# CAREER
# CHA
# F
# NURSES

# CAREER CHANGES FOR NURSES

## WORK OPPORTUNITIES OUTSIDE HOSPITAL

Joanna Lyall

HPL
Hawker Publications

First published in 1993 by
Hawker Publications Ltd
13 Park House
140 Battersea Park Road
London SW11 4NB



British Library Cataloguing in Publication Data

A catalogue record for this book is available from the British Library

ISBN 1 874790 03 5

Designed by
Richard Souper

Typeset by
Hawker Publications Ltd

Printed and bound in Great Britain by
Cox and Wyman, Reading

# CONTENTS

# ACKNOWLEDGEMENTS

I am very grateful to all the nurses who agreed to be interviewed on their personal experience of the occupations outlined in this book.

I would also like to thank Janet Snell and Amanda Tattam of *Nursing Times*, James Buchan, Paul Denton, Pauline Ford, Julia Mountain and the staff of the press office at the Royal College of Nursing. My thanks also to the Institute of Manpower Studies and the library of the King's Fund Centre.

Joanna Lyall is a freelance journalist specialising in health. She has been contributing to *Nursing Times* and *The Health Service Journal* for several years. She has also written for *General Practitioner, Therapy, Which? Way to Health, The Guardian, The Independent* and *Radio Times*. Her previous book, *Living With Cancer*, which she co-authored, won a medical journalism prize.

# INTRODUCTION

Have you ever thought of working on a newspaper, operating a telephone helpline, setting up a clinic, nursing in industry, creating your own job-share arrangement, working your way around the world, establishing a practice in complementary therapies, going into social work or training as a counsellor?

This book is written in the belief that anyone who has trained as a nurse has a great deal to offer, personally and professionally, in a variety of occupations.

We live in changing times, with changing patterns of service, and traditional nursing posts do not always offer the employment security they once promised. But fulfilment can come in many forms, as the nurses interviewed for this book have found. Finding a worthwhile job, temporary or permanent, can often be a matter of research and reflection on your personal preferences, tastes and talent.

The aim of this book is to outline work opportunities you might not previously have considered. For example, we have included practice nursing because it is a new and growing area, but not community nursing or health visiting because these roles will be familiar to every nurse. Our purpose is to give you a flavour of each opportunity, plus essential information to help you decide what would be best for you.

Joanna Lyall, May 1993

# 1 OPPORTUNITIES IN GENERAL PRACTICE

General practice offers nurses the chance of working within a small team, and building up relationships with patients over many years. Hours are fairly regular and there are good opportunities for part-time work.

## Practice nursing

Practice nursing is the fastest growing section of the profession, and, it seems, the happiest. In a survey of 3,000 qualified nurses, published by the Institute of Manpower Studies in October 1992, practice nurses were the most contented with their workload and pay.

A total of 18,000 nurses including part-timers (12,000 whole time equivalents) are now employed in general practice, compared with 8,000 in 1986. This is partly a reflection of the government's policy of shifting resources away from hospitals into the community and a direct result of the new GP contract, introduced on April 1 1990, which lays a much greater emphasis on health promotion, immunisation and screening than was previously the case.

The contract requires GPs or other members of the practice team to provide patients aged 16-74 with health checks (including height, weight and blood pressure) and advice about lifestyle, at least every three years. Patients of 75 and over must be visited at home at least once a year for a general assessment.

The contract also introduced target payments for GPs who reach specified levels of childhood immunisation and cervical cytology. A new sessional fee was introduced for health promotion clinics aimed at diabetes, heart disease, anti-smoking, alcohol control, diet and stress management.

All these factors have led to a rapid increase in the number of nurses employed in general practice and to a

> ***Nikki Cadle,** aged 29, worked as an SEN in Worcestershire for two years and then undertook a 12 month conversion course to SRN at the Whittington Hospital, London. She now works 41 hours a week as a practice nurse at two north London practices.*
>
> **“I like the patient contact you get in practice nursing and the chance to be your own boss. You build up relationships with patients and have a chance to get to know them over a long time. I see the women for antenatals and postnatals and then see the kids for their vaccinations. I was the first practice nurse they had ever had in one of the practices and that gave me a lot of freedom. I started out doing 15 hours and built up.**
>
> **Now I do asthma and diabetes clinics, “well person” checks and heart disease prevention. I’m better paid than I would be in hospital but I’ve also got more responsibility. If I don’t refer someone with high blood pressure to the GP and he goes home and has a heart attack, I’m responsible. There are more opportunities for part-time work and job sharing than in hospitals and the hours are great: no evenings, lates or weekends. My husband works very long hours and I would never see him if I worked in hospital. We hope to start a family soon but I certainly plan to come back to work.”**

widening of their role. Practice nurses are now running asthma, diabetes and epilepsy clinics, undertaking screening of elderly people, running cervical cytology programmes, providing counselling and running minor casualty services. The growing numbers of elderly people in the population means the demand for practice nurses is likely to go on increasing.

The job offers flexibility, a fair amount of autonomy, many part-time opportunities and the chance to work with a small team. Many find the absence of a management structure one of the most appealing aspects of working in general practice. The practice nurse can have a considerable input into the running and organisation of the group. And despite the high rate of patient turnover in some areas, general practice still offers continuity of care and the possibility of looking after patients over many years. It also offers regular hours and free weekends.

**Training:** No specialist training is required but the English National Board (ENB) Practice Nurse course is available at more than 40 centres. It involves a minimum of 10 days and includes management and techniques for the treatment room. Details from the ENB Resources and Careers section.

**Pay:** By negotiation with individual practices; influenced by how much the local Family Health Service Authority will reimburse. Pay usually £6.36-£10.62 an hour.

**Holidays:** 4-5 weeks.

# Practice management

Initiative, personnel skills, ability to plan ahead, enthusiasm, boundless energy and a sense of humour are some of the attributes called for in advertisements for practice managers. And there is no shortage of applicants. Vacancies often attract between 30 and 60 candidates.

The role and recognition of practice managers has increased greatly over the last ten years with the growing emphasis on business skills, greater computerisation, and the advent of the GP fundholding scheme which gives participating practices their own budgets.

But despite the many recent changes and the growing

acceptance of teamwork in primary care, GPs remain self-employed, independent contractors and they can take time to recognise the benefits of allowing someone else to run part of their business. Diplomacy and flexibility, and acceptance that you cannot change things overnight, are essential for anyone considering this job, according to experienced practice managers.

The advantages include regular hours, the opportunity to work within a small group and make a considerable contribution to the success of the practice.

The practice manager has a key role in maintaining good relations between the GPs and staff. The job also includes interviewing and employing staff, organising the appointments system and PAYE, overseeing record keeping, filling in quarterly returns for the Family Health Service Authority and submitting target figures, drawing up a business plan, familiarising GP trainees with practice management, and organising clinics and practice meetings.

**Pay:** By negotiation with individual practices. Whitley Council staff rates range from £9,837 to £28,364 according to the responsibility involved.

**Training:** A course leading to the Diploma in Practice Management, established by the Association of Medical Secretaries, Practice Administrators and Receptionists (AMSPAR), is available at more than 50 colleges around the country. The course, available on a half-day and day release basis, requires at least 240 hours of study over not more than two academic years. It covers management of general practice, legal aspects of practice administration, premises, communication, finance skills, data processing and research. The course fees are generally met by the practice, with part or all of the cost then reimbursed by the Family Health Service Authority.

The Association of Health Centre and Practice Administrators (AHCPA) also offers training leading to a Diploma in Practice Management. The course is offered at

*Jenny Ridge, aged 40, trained at the London Hospital, Whitechapel and was a ward sister at St Mary's Roehampton, before she left to go into general practice as a nurse/receptionist in 1979. She became practice manager in 1990. The practice in Roehampton has 6,000 patients, three doctors, a GP trainee, three nurse/receptionists, a part-time secretary, computer operator and part-time finance officer. Jenny is responsible for recruiting staff, organising the rotas, claiming payments, ordering drugs and organising health promotion clinics.*

**“I like the variety of practice management – you're responsible for everything from the loo rolls to the plumbing – and the satisfaction of things going smoothly. We are hitting our targets and I find that very worthwhile. I also enjoy the patient contact. I said I wanted to continue some nursing when I was made practice manager, and I still spend about 40 per cent of my time seeing patients and running clinics. We do asthma, hypertension, and "well woman" clinics as well as assessments of elderly people. I love the patient contact and the family aspect of general practice.**

**As a practice manager you need diplomacy and flexibility. Having a nursing background helps because it teaches you how to get on with people. We get on very well as a team and there is no "them and us" divide between doctors and staff that you get in some practices. But I do find it difficult if I ever have to discipline the staff, or the doctors. That is the hardest part of the job. And the time pressures are horrible. You have to structure your time carefully.”**

a handful of colleges around the country. Topics covered include communications, business plans, managing a budget, cash flow analysis, identifying staff needs and managing meetings. **Holidays:** 4-6 weeks.

# 2 OCCUPATIONAL HEALTH NURSING

Occupational health (OH) nursing is concerned with the health of people at work and their working environment. Of some 8,000 OH nurses in the UK, about three quarters work in factories, offices and other commercial organisations.

In the private sector, OH nurses are expected to understand the pressures of the marketplace, and prove their own worth in developing an efficient workforce.

Company managers tend to judge occupational health only in terms of reduction in accidents or absenteeism; they may be reluctant to introduce or expand services for which they see no obvious or immediate benefit. So OH nurses need to be good at making contacts, adept at putting across the needs of individual workers, prepared to fight their corner and put up a convincing case for anything they propose. "Not a job for shrinking violets" as one OH nurse commented.

You must also be able to react quickly, and be competent and confident working on your own, as many organisations employ only one nurse. But if you enjoy autonomy and like the idea of investigating all aspects of a working environment, the job offers considerable scope.

You need to communicate well with all levels – managers, staff and union representatives – and build up trust. You must also keep abreast with health and safety legislation.

In addition to providing regular clinics, which enable staff to be seen "in house" rather than taking time off to see their GP, OH nurses carry out pre-employment health assessments, provide emergency treatment, teach first aid and offer counselling and support for employees with

***Christine Mitchell**, aged 51, has been in charge of occupational health at The Guardian and Manchester Evening News (where she is the only nurse) for the past eight years. Based in Manchester where she holds daily clinics for all staff, she spends three days a month in London visiting the printing plant on the Isle of Dogs as well as the Guardian office. She also trains staff in first aid. She did her nurse training at the Manchester Royal Infirmary and previously worked in neurology. She has a certificate in occupational health nursing.*

**“ I got into occupational health almost by accident: I was at home looking after the children, then needed a job when my husband was made redundant. Now it's my favourite branch of medicine. You have a chance of getting to know people in their working context and the time to establish a rapport. But you have to be self-sufficient, able to work on your own and confident in your clinical decisions. There's no one I can discuss patients with. It is also important to understand all the jobs and the equipment people work with.**

**You also need to be assertive, be able to communicate with all levels of people, and stand up for what patients need. They're very good to me here but in occupational health you are always at the mercy of the company. It can be frustrating if you can't persuade them to pay for equipment which you know would benefit staff. There is always more you would like to do. And it's difficult to prove our effectiveness. But very satisfying when, for example, you persuade someone to lose weight, stop smoking and bring down their blood pressure. ”**

problems. They assess the working environment for potential hazards, looking at equipment, lifting practice, furniture, floors, heating and lighting. They also organise general screening, health promotion clinics, pre-retirement

***Jean Raper**, aged 56, has been in occupational health for 30 years. She has worked in the iron and steel industries, potteries, construction sites and trawlers. She is now Chief Occupational Nurse with Sheffield City Council which employs 27,000 people. With eight other nurses she is responsible for running routine clinics, carrying out statutory medicals and assessing employees' fitness following accident or injury.*

*She and her team also run menopause, PMT (premenstrual tension) and immunisation clinics, and provide training sessions to help disabled employees integrate into the workforce. They have also run Tai Chi sessions. She is chairman of the RCN's Society of Occupational Health Nurses.*

**“ I like the autonomy of the job and the scope for innovation. Most occupational health nurses work alone and you must be accountable for everything you do. It is not a job for someone who requires a lot of peer group support. You must be able to communicate with all types of people at all levels of an organisation, and be prepared to sell your message. Most people know about healthy living, and when they're rocking the boat, but need to be persuaded to accept lifestyle changes.**

**I see my role as enabler rather than enforcer. Tact and diplomacy are always needed. Having to persuade a manager to be sympathetic to an employee who is not pulling their weight can be difficult without breaking confidentiality. It is also upsetting when someone is no longer fit for their job and can't be offered an alternative.**

**You must be prepared to go wherever the employees are working, see what their health needs are and how you can help them. I hated going to the abattoir to look at the work of the meat inspectors. But it is satisfying to help people overcome their problems and get back to work. Seventy of the 72 people referred with alcohol problems last year are now back at work. ”**

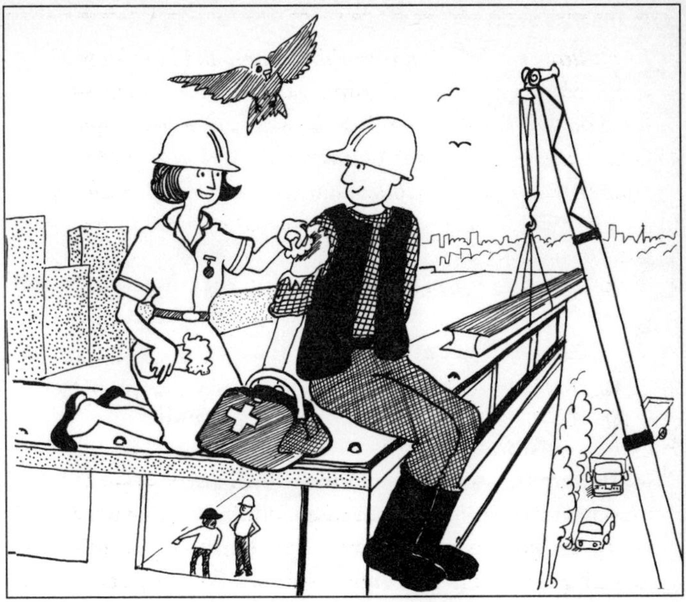
Eve Morris

*You must be prepared to go wherever the employees are working.*

screening, fitness assessments and referrals to specialists, GPs, opticians, voluntary agencies and support groups. Some OH departments, both NHS and private, provide a service for other organisations as a way of bringing in extra income. And some OH companies have been established to serve a number of clients on a contract basis.

**Pay:** £12,000 - £22,000 in the NHS
Occupational Health Adviser, Post Office – £18,749 - £22,707
OH Nurse, Oil company, Cheshire – £17,000.

**Holidays:** 5-6 weeks.

**Training:** Specialist training is not mandatory to work as an OH nurse. About a dozen colleges offer a course (one year full time or two years part time) leading to a Diploma in Occupational Health Nursing. A degree course is also available. Details from the English National Board.

# 3 NURSING IN SCHOOLS

School nurses are responsible for carrying out health interviews when children start school, and checking each child's growth, sight and hearing. They discuss the management of any problems with parents and teachers and advise on the care of children with conditions such as diabetes or asthma.

School nurses also give health education talks, check immunisations and provide counselling for children and parents. In cases of suspected child abuse they become involved in case conferences. They no longer carry out routine hair inspections but still advise on the prevention and treatment of head lice.

In boarding schools, nurses are responsible for providing 24-hour care, treatment of injuries, and organisation of GP surgeries. They are responsible for pupils admitted to the sanatorium, and also provide pastoral care.

School nurses have the opportunity to get to know children over several years and build up relationships with parents and teachers. They can play a very important part in ensuring children with special needs are integrated into the school population and get the best from their education. They also have an important health education role, explaining issues such as healthy eating, exercise, smoking, sexuality, and alcohol abuse. The job requires good social skills and an empathy with children.

It can be suitable for those with school-age children of their own, who want to spend time with them during the holidays. But not all school nurses have school holidays free. Others are employed, and paid, in term time only.

***Mary Abraham,** aged 60, went into school nursing ten years ago after she was made redundant from her job as occupational health manager for a hotel group. She is a school nurse in South West London, responsible for five inner city primary schools with a population of 1,100. She is also chairman of the RCN's School Nurses Forum.*

**“ The most enjoyable part of school nursing is the contact with children and parents, developing care plans and seeing children improve and progress. The worst part of the job is the lack of space. You may have to do hearing tests in a corridor and some school nurses have had to do eye tests in the playground.**

**Ten years ago the role of the school nurse was very much lining children up and checking for vermin. Now we are much more concerned with health promotion and individual needs. We don't do routine medicals on all children but invite the parents of new pupils for health interviews, and then agree a care plan if there are any problems. The parents may be very concerned about a problem such as bedwetting, and we can reassure them and explain what help is available. Educating teachers about how to treat children suffering from diabetes, epilepsy or asthma is also part of our role.**

**The sadistic PE teacher is a thing of the past, but some staff still need educating on the importance of asthmatic children being able to use their inhalers whenever they need to. As a school nurse you need to be realistic as well as tactful. Elaborate healthy eating advice is no good to a family living in a bed and breakfast. Ten years ago school nurses were looked down on by health visitors and other nursing colleagues and seen very much as assistants to school doctors. Things have improved since then but I would still like to see a mandatory specialist training for school nurses. ”**

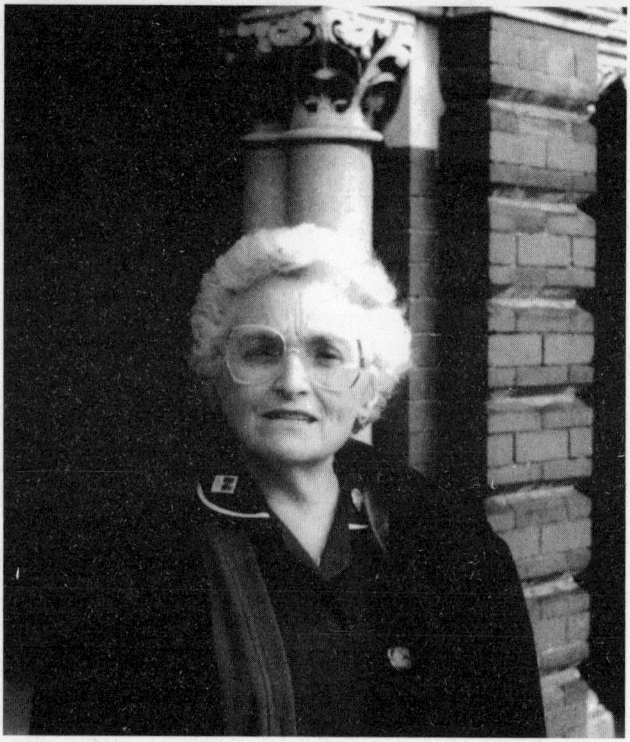

***Marilyn Watts, aged 56,*** *is sister-in-charge at Marlborough College, Wiltshire, which has 600 boys and 300 girls, and 100 teaching staff. With two full and three part-time nurses she provides 24-hour cover seven days a week.*

*Her previous experience includes home care for the dying, and nursing in a community hospital. She is an executive committee member of the Boarding Schools Association.*

**“ I never expected to be a school nurse but I love it. You get very involved and there is a lot of pastoral work, advising on relationships, work crises and eating disorders. I like getting to know the pupils and seeing them go right through the school.**

**The local GP holds a surgery here six days a week and we help run that as well as routine medicals for all the new pupils. There are over 5,000 visits per term to the sanatorium and we admit about 200 per term.**

**There are a lot of sports injuries and we do some of the suturing and plastering, and make the dental guards for rugby and hockey. We also do all the immunisations for pupils going overseas. In term time I work 65-90 hours a week, including on-call time, and sleep in the school two or three nights a week. There is a lot of contact with parents and housemasters; you need to be a good communicator.**

**Independent schools are extremely tough employers and it's important to get the contract, terms of service and hours in writing before you start. A lot of independent school nurses are on call every night. The accommodation is often appalling and only available during the term time.**

**All schools expect total involvement and it's important to be able to present yourself well and not allow yourself to be treated as inferior. There is a tendency to look on anyone without a degree as a second class citizen. In the past, nursing in independent schools has been poorly understood and lacked status. Things are improving but some still think of matron counting the socks. ”**

**Pay:** Most school nurses employed by health authorities earn £13,750-£16,830 (F grade, £7.00 to £8.60 an hour). Those in independent schools earn £8,000-£18,000.

**Holidays** range from five weeks to full school holidays.

**Training:** No specialist training is required to work as a school nurse but a 12-week course leading to the School Nurse's Certificate is available at more than 20 colleges. Details from the English National Board.

# 4 WORKING FOR A NURSING AGENCY

Nursing agencies operate in most parts of the UK and offer opportunities for those interested in management as well as hands-on nursing work, full time or part time. Nursing agencies also offer RGNs the chance of working from home, providing an on-call telephone advice service for patients and the agency's nurses, in case of emergency. All nursing agencies are required by law to provide this 24-hour service.

## Agency nursing

Working as an agency nurse can offer variety, flexible hours, a chance to broaden your experience without committing yourself to a full-time job, and employment at short notice. The opportunities will vary, according to your availability, geographical location and experience, but working for an agency is a good option for those who want to choose exactly when and how much they work. It may also be the right way of working if your home commitments are very variable.

Agency nursing can help you re-adjust after a period abroad and can be a good choice when you are between jobs, trying to decide where your next career move should take you. An agency may point you in a direction you had not previously considered. One with a national network of branches will know about general trends and opportunities outside your immediate locality.

You need to be reliable, flexible and extremely adaptable,

***Sue Gray**, aged 41, is the British Nursing Association's area manager for the South East of England, in charge of 19 branches and some 50 staff. She trained at the Westminster group of hospitals and worked on a surgical ward and as a district nurse before joining an agency after the birth of her son.*

**“ I went into agency work because it was convenient and allowed me to keep up my connection with nursing. I was a branch assistant then branch manager before being promoted to area manager in 1984. You need to be self-motivated to succeed in agency work and really want to see the business expand. It is office hours, Monday to Friday, but it's not an easy option. It's as pressurised as working on a ward, although the pressures are not physical. You need to be able to think and work fast.**

**I like the variety and the satisfaction of getting new clients. About half my time is spent out of the office, visiting clients. You need to keep abreast of the health market and identify needs. A few years ago 70 per cent of our business was from the NHS, now it's only 40 per cent with the rest coming from the private sector. Working on the administration side of an agency demands good interpersonal and organisation skills, and commercial awareness. You are responsible for interviewing staff, assessing clients, general administration, making sure clients are billed, and collecting debts. I'm also responsible for teaching branch staff. ”**

able to pick up different procedures and practices quickly and ready to accept that there is more than one way of doing things. Extremely good social skills are also important as you are likely to be meeting new patients and staff all the time. If you are working in the patient's own home you should be prepared to fit in with the individual's routines and habits, and be adept at assessing family situations. (Almost half the placements made by the British Nursing Association are for home nursing). You may also have to fit into a group which includes other, non-nursing, staff. Tact is important.

## Agency management

Nursing agencies also employ large numbers of nurses on the office side as branch managers, responsible for visiting clients and assessing their needs, interviewing and placing nurses, office management, budgets and record keeping.

This is a job for those who are keen to keep up with the care side of nursing but also want the challenge of running a commercially successful operation.

You need to be efficient, good under pressure, able to keep abreast of developments in the health care market, capable of expanding the business and delivering a profit. Time management and good interviewing skills are essential, and you should be a good judge of people, to ensure successful placements. Secretarial skills are also useful.

Area managers have overall responsibility for all the branches in their patch and spend a lot of time on the road, building up new business as well as visiting the local offices.

**Pay:** Agency nurses are generally paid the mid-point of the grade for the job. Agencies deduct national insurance and tax, unless you are working in the patient's own home, in which case you are considered self-employed.
Branch Managers: £12,400-£14,400
Area Managers: £20,000-£24,000

**Holidays:** Branch staff – 4-5 weeks.

# 5 WORKING IN THE PHARMACEUTICAL INDUSTRY

The UK pharmaceutical industry has an annual turnover of some £7billion, employs more than 70,000 people and spends some £90million a year on research. Drug companies offer good working conditions, opportunities for career progression and fairly regular hours. There are also opportunities for part-time work. The industry accords importance to training and individual development. Many companies operate performance-related pay schemes and company cars are usually offered.

Many of the drug companies are concentrated in the south east of England. There are, however, opportunities in independent clinical research organisations, which carry out projects for pharmaceutical companies, in other parts of the UK.

To succeed in the industry you need an interest in pharmacology and research, good presentational skills and self-assurance. Appearance is also important - each employee is seen as a representative of the company. You also need to appreciate the demands of working in a commercial environment.

Nurses are at an advantage because of their knowledge of physiology and pharmacology, their inter-personal skills, their understanding of the NHS and experience of working with doctors.

There are opportunities for nurses as:

- **Medical Representative**, promoting drugs or products to GPs and hospital doctors
- **Clinical Research Associate** (also known as Clinical Research Scientist) responsible for setting up and

overseeing Phase 2, 3 and 4 clinical research trials on patients in hospitals and general practice

- **Clinical Research Nurse**, looking after healthy volunteers taking part in Phase 1 clinical trials
- **Nurse Adviser**, advising GPs and practice nurses on setting up clinics in areas such as asthma, diabetes and hypertension, in which the drug company has an interest.

*Katy Jones, aged 31, has been a medical rep with Glaxo since 1987, working in the fields of gastroenterology, antibiotics, dermatology and migraine. Before joining the company, she completed a psychology degree, did research at the London Hospital on health care in the East End, then trained as a nurse at St George's Hospital, London.*

**“ You need to be a self-starter as a rep and continually self-motivated. All reps write their own business plan and take responsibility for meeting targets. It's important to be commercially aware. You also need to be able to work on your own. Confidence is important but that grows with experience. Being a nurse improves your credibility with doctors, and your understanding of how the NHS works is helpful.**

**The job involves promoting pharmaceutical products to GPs, hospital doctors and pharmacists. In a day I might see three GPs, one or two hospital doctors and two pharmacists. Some GPs like to see reps before surgery so I generally work eight to five. But it can be later if I have to organise an evening meeting for GPs to meet consultants. There is also quite a lot of paperwork. We log what we do each day.**

**It's a very different culture from the NHS and less stressful than working on a ward. I find it challenging and like being part of a career structure. You are treated very much as an individual. ”**

Drug companies see the nurse adviser's role as primarily educational and not promotional. There are also opportunities for nurses in the pharmaceutical companies' regulatory affairs and adverse reactions departments.

## Medical Representative

Medical "reps" are drug companies' sales force although their targets – GPs, hospital doctors and pharmacists – do not actually buy anything from them. The job is to promote prescription of your company's products by making sure they are known about and understood.

Medical reps call on practices and hospitals within an assigned area, by appointment, and discuss any new research results related to their product. They also organise large meetings of GPs and consultants.

Drug reps are drawn from a variety of backgrounds and not all have degrees or a professional qualification. But nurses are at an advantage because of their training and their knowledge of the NHS and its professional groups. Companies provide training in the therapeutic area in which you will be working and the drugs involved, and in selling skills – including practice sessions with a video.

The job requires self-reliance as you will be out on the road alone much of the time and may sometimes have to wait an hour or more before you can see the doctor. You must also be prepared for rebuffs. Some doctors think seeing reps is very far down the list of priorities. The challenge is to get in there and build up a positive reception for yourself, your company and your product.

## Clinical Research Nurse

As a a Clinical Research Nurse you will be working in a clinical pharmacology unit, looking after healthy adult volunteers who are taking part in Phase 1 clinical trials.

Units usually have 10-20 beds and are similar to intensive care units with one nurse for every patient. The volunteers are sometimes drawn from the drug company's staff. Some companies have clinical research units in hospitals.

Clinical Research Nurses are responsible for organising preliminary medicals for all potential volunteers, followed by another medical just before the study.

The work on the unit can be quite intensive, with nurses carrying out hourly ECGs and blood pressure checks, and in the case of intravenous infusions blood may be taken every few minutes during the first hour.

The units generally work a five day week but the days can be long, from 7am to 6.30pm in some cases. Some pharmaceutical companies also employ nurses as bank staff for their clinical pharmacology units.

Some Clinical Research Nurse jobs ask for at least two years post-registration experience, and if you have experience in a hi-tech area such as ITU or cardiac care, it is an advantage.

The work is very different from hospital nursing as the "patients" are healthy volunteers, usually only in for 24 hours. And the focus, of course, is on research rather than helping people back to recovery. But the job offers the interest, and satisfaction, of being in on the early stages of a new drug or formulation.

## Clinical Research Associate

Clinical Research Associates are responsible for designing, setting up and monitoring clinical research trials involving hospitals and GP practices. This includes drawing up the protocol for the study, liaising with ethics committees and regulatory bodies, meeting doctors to outline the proposed study, persuading them to become involved, and overseeing and monitoring the data collection.

The work demands a thorough knowledge of the

***Sue Miller, aged 44,*** *trained at the Central Middlesex Hospital, and has worked in occupational health and a plastic surgery unit. She is now a Senior Clinical Research Scientist (CRS) with Glaxo, responsible for setting up clinical trials in hospitals and general practice all over the UK.*

**❝ Sixty per cent of the work of a CRS is out and about visiting GPs, hospital consultants, pharmacy departments and haematology labs. There is a great deal of travelling involved; I drive about 30,000 miles a year. The remaining time is spent on designing the trial, interaction between the various departments involved, and administration.**

**The skills needed for the job are stamina, diplomacy and organisation. You also need to know your therapeutic area very thoroughly, as you must be able to talk to consultants at their own level. You build up good working relationships and are treated very much as an equal.**

**You need to be a self-starter – it is up to the CRS to determine how the trial should proceed. There is a high degree of responsibility. In a gastroenterology trial, for example, you may be co-ordinating a study with as many as 100 centres taking part. You need to be meticulous about detail, and good record keeping is essential. Every telephone call and trip to a centre must be written up.**

**There is a lot of liaison within the company, with sales staff, statistics and packaging departments. The job also involves contact with the Committee on Safety of Medicines, ethics committees and regional health authorities. A nursing background is useful because you have a good grounding in various therapeutic areas, and understand the environment in which you are working. You work hard in a pharmaceutical company, and are rewarded for the results you achieve. I enjoy the mental stimulation and the constant challenge of the job. ❞**

therapeutic area concerned, good communication skills, organisational ability and strong attention to detail. You need to be numerate and analytical. The job is likely to involve a lot of travel.

## Nurse Adviser

Since the introduction of the general practitioners' new contract with its stress on health promotion, and the introduction of a new sessional fee for GPs running diabetes and heart disease clinics, drug companies have turned more attention to employing nurses to provide support and advice for practices in specific therapeutic areas.

Nurse Advisers provide educational material for patients and advise practice nurses and GPs about setting up special clinics for asthma, diabetes and hypertension. This area of employment seems likely to increase because of the government's emphasis on prevention, and the drive to reduce deaths from strokes and heart disease.

There are also specialist nurses employed by pharmaceutical companies as incontinence and stoma care advisers. There are some opportunities for part-time and temporary work.

**Pay:**
Medical Representative – £12,000-£30,000 including bonuses, plus car
Clinical Research Nurse – £14,000-£19,000
Clinical Research Associate – £14,000-£30,000 plus car
Nurse Adviser – £16,000-£20,000

**Holidays:** 4-5 weeks.

# 6 ALLIED THERAPIES: COUNSELLING, CHIROPODY, PHYSIOTHERAPY, SOCIAL WORK

Careers such as counselling, chiropody, physiotherapy and social work offer considerable contact with people and a chance to work with patients and clients on a one to one basis. They also offer jobs in a variety of settings including hospitals, general practice, private practice, industry and the community.

While nurses may be at an advantage when applying for training because of their proven interpersonal skills, competition for places in some areas – physiotherapy for example – is intense.

## Counselling

Counselling can offer valuable help in a range of distressing situations from job stress, redundancy and bereavement, to major disasters and marriage breakdown. There are counsellors working in newspaper offices, hospitals, universities, GP surgeries, industry, charities and schools. Many counsellors work from home as private practitioners.

Interest in counselling and what it can offer has increased substantially in recent years. The British Association for Counselling (BAC), founded in 1977, has some 9,500 individuals and 500 organisations in membership. The BAC also has a special Counselling in Medical Settings group.

Counselling is a process involving clarification, discussion and, ideally, resolution of distressing issues and situations. The BAC defines it as "the skilled and principled use of relationship to facilitate self-knowledge, emotional

***Meg Barham, aged 48,*** *has been a counsellor at Thomas's Hospital, London since 1984, and now heads a team of four, providing a counselling service for some 7,500 staff. She was previously Senior Nursing Officer at Northwick Park Hospital. She trained at Paddington General Hospital and has worked in Holland and Western Canada, where she cared for Cree Indians. She is a BAC accredited counsellor; her training included a three-year counselling diploma course at South West London College, which she undertook on a part-time basis while nursing at night. She is a founder member of the National Association for Staff Support, a charity established in 1988 to promote better support for NHS staff.*

**“ The best part of my job is being able to give people space, to see them grow and gain insight. Spending time talking to patients was what I most enjoyed in nursing.**

**People in the health service are enormously committed but the support for them is often abysmal. And the level of denial is enormous. Counselling allows staff to say they feel sad, stressed and anxious. The bulk of the work is concerned with relationships but people also come with alcohol problems, bereavement and depression. Sometimes they come with a work-related difficulty but work is not usually the main problem.**

**We get about 120 new referrals a year and the largest part of our work is with nurses. Being a nurse, and having spent 30 years in the health service, helps me understand the organisational and professional issues which are very important.**

**I think you need sensitivity and a good sense of humour as a counsellor. You must be committed and motivated, as training and ongoing supervision are very expensive. Counselling is more reflective than nursing and not task-orientated. Understanding of its value is growing but there is still a long way to go. Only a handful of NHS hospitals provide a service for staff. ”**

acceptance and growth, and the optimal development of personal resources". Clients should leave feeling happier, stronger and better able to cope. The basic values of counselling, according to the BAC, are integrity, impartiality and respect. Emphasis is also placed on the client's right to self-determination: "Counsellors do not normally give advice" says BAC's Code of Practice.

**Training**

There is nothing to stop anyone setting up as a counsellor. Unlike doctors and nurses, counsellors are not subject to a regulatory body such as the UKCC (United Kingdom Central Council for Nursing, Midwifery and Health Visiting) or the doctors' General Medical Council, which lay down statutory training and registration requirements. There is no mandatory training for counsellors.

However there are moves to introduce some regulation into the counselling world. BAC has introduced systems for accrediting individual counsellors and counselling courses. Most of the courses it recognises are for one year's full-time study, or two to three years part time, involving a minimum of 450 hours training and study.

This is the sort of preparation necessary to become a counsellor, BAC maintains. Shorter "counselling skills" courses are not usually designed to train people as counsellors, it adds. BAC publishes a directory of training courses in counselling and psychotherapy, which includes entry requirements.

In order to be accredited by BAC, individual counsellors must have completed at least 450 hours of training, and 450 hours of counselling practice, under supervision. Those who have not undergone formal training must provide evidence of ten years' experience in counselling, with a minimum of 150 hours per year under supervision. Applicants for accreditation must also have an ongoing arrangement for supervision. There are more than 600 BAC accredited counsellors.

**Code of Practice**

BAC has published a Code of Ethics and Practice for Counsellors which all its members must agree to. This covers matters such as confidentiality, advertising and contracting with clients. The code states, among other things, that counsellors should work in ways which promote the client's control over his/her life, and should not exploit clients financially, sexually or emotionally. "Engaging in sexual activity with current clients or within 12 weeks of the end of the counselling relationship is unethical," according to the code. Where there has been a long professional relationship a lifetime prohibition on any sexual relationship may be more appropriate, it adds. The code also specifies that all counsellors should be undergoing supervision themselves and should not counsel when their own functioning is impaired through emotional difficulties, illness, alcohol or drugs.

Counselling requires a wide-ranging interest in people, sensitivity, good concentration and patience. It may be weeks, or even months, for the counselling process to achieve results, and clients can direct a fair amount of hostility to the counsellor along the way. Maturity and life experience are important. It is undoubtedly very satisfying to work with individuals at quite a deep level but you must be realistic about what counselling can achieve. And the autonomy of the counsellor could be frightening, at least initially, for those used to working in a team.

You should also be at ease working one to one for most of the time and yet be able to stand up for your department, or role, within the organisation. Counsellors are relatively recent arrivals in hospitals, general practices and business organisations, and are not automatically accorded the status of other professional groups.

**Pay:**

Counsellors in NHS – £10,000-£20,000
Counsellor in training, university – £9,000

Drug counsellor, advice project – £17,814
Counsellor/trainer, regional alcohol project – £14,106
Private Practice – £15-£40 per 50min session.

Jobs are advertised in *The Guardian, The Independent,* and in specialist publications such as the *Times Educational Supplement* and the *Times Higher Education Supplement.*

# Chiropody

Chiropodists diagnose and treat foot diseases and disorders such as corns, verrucae, callouses, fungal infections of the toenails and advise on appliances, and specialist shoes. They also carry out minor surgery. Job opportunities are good and seem likely to increase to meet the needs of an expanding elderly population.

Chiropodists work in hospitals, community clinics, GP practices, industry, offices and private practice. There are also some domiciliary services. There are opportunities to work part time, and some chiropodists combine private practice and NHS sessions.

### Training

In order to work in the NHS as a chiropodist you must be state registered. This requires a three year full-time training at one of the 14 recognised colleges in the UK, leading to a BSc degree in Podiatry. The entrance requirement is generally two A-levels, but an RGN qualification would usually be accepted as equivalent. The course covers anatomy, physiology, pathology, orthopaedics, bacteriology, chemistry, physiotherapy and local anaesthesia. A high proportion of the training is practical; it includes treatment of patients under the supervision of experienced chiropodists, and the preparation of appliances. There is however no requirement for chiropodists in private practice to be state registered.

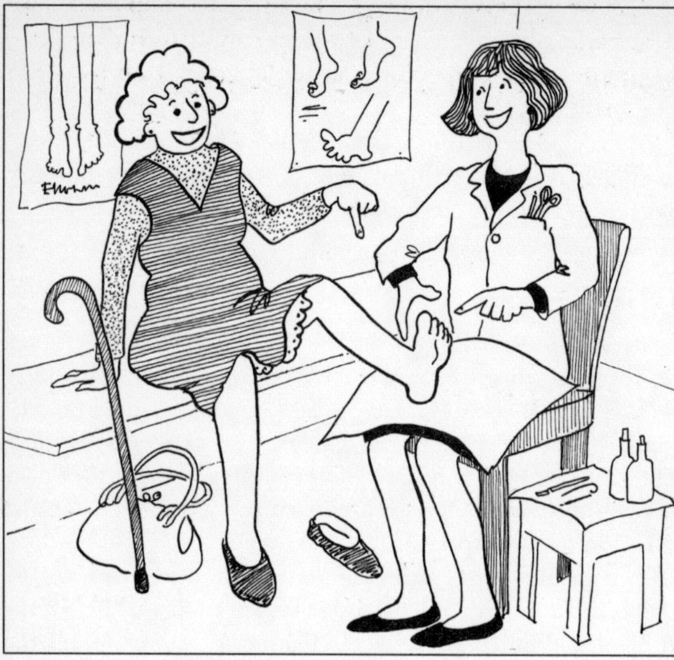

Eve Morris

*It helps if you enjoy working with elderly people...*

Chiropody requires dexterity, a liking for people, an easy manner and an even temperament. You may see 16-20 patients a day in NHS clinics, and possibly more if you work in private practice.

You should be able to put people at their ease, and inspire confidence. It helps if you enjoy working with elderly people, as a high proportion of patients comes from that group. Success in private practice will also require some marketing skills and good local contacts.

Chiropodists are responsible for diagnosis as well as treatment, and have the right to treat patients without direction or referral from a doctor. And they are responsible for certain surgical treatments under local anaesthesia. So the job involves a fair amount of autonomy.

Private practice can offer good financial rewards, and the

satisfaction of running your own business. Start-up costs can be substantial however: £4,000-£7,000 including an automatic treatment chair, autoclave, drill and other equipment.

**Pay :**
NHS chiropodist – £13,300 - £18,100
District chief chiropodist – £26,500
Private practice – £10-£25 per half-hour treatment

**Holidays:** 6 weeks.

# Physiotherapy

A career in physiotherapy offers secure prospects in a variety of settings. The NHS has been short of up to 1,000 physiotherapists for several years, according to the Chartered Society of Physiotherapy.

In addition to NHS posts in hospital and the community there are also opportunities to work in commercial organisations and private practice. There are also opportunities to specialise in outpatient work, paediatrics, the treatment of strokes, sports injuries and hydrotherapy.

Physiotherapy requires an interest in rehabilitation, facility for working as part of a team, physical fitness and good communication skills. An interest in sport and physical education is an advantage. A personality which inspires confidence and optimism is also an asset.

### Training

Training is a three year full-time course leading to a BSc in Physiotherapy which entitles the holder to state registration. There are some three dozen colleges in the UK offering approved courses. Details are available from the Chartered Society of Physiotherapy. There are also some four year honours degree courses.

Entry requirements are generally five GCSEs and two A

levels, but colleges will consider other qualifications. Mature applicants are viewed favourably and about a third of all UK students are over 21 when they begin training.

The training includes anatomy, psychology, general pathology, medicine and surgery, manipulative procedures and thermal and electrical treatments as they relate to therapy. At least 1,000 hours of clinical practice are undertaken as part of the course.

**Pay:**
Starting salary NHS – £11,500
Senior Physiotherapist – £13,300-£18,000
District Physiotherapist – £27,400
Private practice per half-hour session – £19-£30

# Social work

Social work requires practical common sense and broad life experience, as well as empathy and the ability to build up rapport with a wide range of people. It is not a career for the rigid or judgemental, or those who like to see swift results from their interventions. While some clients may be helped over a crisis, or sudden change in circumstances, in one or two sessions, many will require much longer-term support for a variety of practical and emotional difficulties.

In some cases the social worker's role is to help the client come to terms with very difficult and immutable circumstances, such as permanent disability or chronic illness, and this can involve a great deal of anger and resentment on the client's part.

The job requires resilience and objectivity. And broad shoulders. Social workers, unlike nurses, are seen in a negative light by many people and do not get a good press. Their day-to-day work seems to go largely unsung while any miscalculation, such as a failure to remove a child from what prove to be violent parents, is likely to be widely publicised. There can be great satisfaction in relieving

***Grainne Murray, aged 30,** trained as an RGN at Guy's Hospital and worked in a hospice before undertaking social work training. She completed a four year degree course in Social Work, which included the Certificate of Qualification in Social Work, at Middlesex Polytechnic, with a local authority grant. She has been a social worker specialising in oncology at St Bartholomew's hospital since 1991.*

**“ I loved nursing but realised I was most interested in the psychosocial aspects of caring for patients. In some ways there is more mileage in social work and greater variety. I advise on financial problems and the benefits system, organise discharges, make referrals to local social service departments, occupational therapists, home care services, nursing homes and hospices. A lot of my time is spent providing emotional support, counselling and helping people to adjust to change. People affected by cancer can be very distressed.**

**Because I have autonomy I can spend a lot of time with people who have emotional difficulties, and I find that satisfying. It is also satisfying to be able to mobilise help for patients. But it is not as easy as in nursing to feel part of a ward team. And it can be difficult to go up to a patient on a ward and start making a relationship, particularly if he or she does not want to be seen as in need of social work support. As a nurse you have a physical task to do, so it's much easier.**

**I'm very lucky to be part of a well staffed department – 19 social workers in all. But social work has an uncertain status, especially in hospitals, and you have to prove yourself again and again. Doctors and nurses tend to look for instant results and do not understand that some of the problems brought to a head by illness may have been developing for 20 years or so and cannot always be solved. ”**

anxiety and helping clients manage and improve their circumstances. But your help and skills may not be widely acknowledged as some people still associate seeing a social worker with fecklessness and failure. It is not an easy job and requires considerable maturity and realism, and the ability to recognise your own limitations.

Social workers operate from a variety of settings including hospitals, local authority social services departments, health centres, schools, child guidance clinics and charities. Employment opportunities are good although the level of recruitment is affected by the level of public expenditure.

**Training**

The main qualification for social workers is the Diploma in Social Work (DipSW) which involves training on a two year full-time (or three year part-time) course, approved by the Central Council for Education and Training in Social Work (CCETSW). There are some 130 centres in UK offering an approved course (details from CCETSW). Areas covered include public administration, law and ethical issues, and the course includes supervised practice and assessment.

Applicants under 21 are generally required to have 2 A levels and three GCSEs. Candidates aged 21 and over are not required to have formal educational qualifications but colleges "look for evidence of an ability to study at advanced level", according to CCETSW. Mature applicants are welcomed by colleges.

Social work offers opportunities for part-time and locum work. Jobs are advertised in *The Guardian* newspaper and *Community Care* magazine.

**Pay:**

Social Worker – £12,438-£18,231
Senior Social Worker/team leader – £19,110-£21,462
Director of Social Work Services,
Special Hospital – £27,824

**Holidays:** 5-6 weeks.

# 7 WORKING IN COMPLEMENTARY THERAPIES

Interest in complementary therapies has increased greatly in the last decade, among the public and orthodox health professionals alike. And consumers' use of non-orthodox treatments looks likely to go on increasing.

A survey published by *Which?* in November 1992 found one in four readers visited a complementary practitioner each year, almost double the proportion who were doing so in 1986. The therapies most often used were osteopathy, chiropractic, homeopathy, acupuncture, aromatherapy, reflexology and herbalism.

A MORI survey in 1989 showed three out of four people believed complementary therapies should be available on the NHS, and the Department of Health (DoH) appears to have taken note. In December 1991 guidance from the DoH said GPs could employ complementary practitioners in their practice, providing the doctors remained clinically responsible for the care offered by the therapist.

Many hospitals and hospices are now introducing some complementary therapies such as therapeutic massage, reflexology and aromatherapy as part of routine care. The RCN's Complementary Therapies Special Interest Group, established in 1991, has approaching 1,000 members and has drawn up guidance on training courses.

There is no state register of complementary practitioners and no umbrella organisation setting national standards or accrediting training courses. There are, however, federations and membership organisations within the individual therapies, which have a regulatory function. Some therapies have five or more such organisations.

Anyone considering a training course should do careful research and find out about the validity of any qualification offered. Guidance from the RCN's Complementary Therapies Special Interest Group lists the following points to consider:

Is the course validated by any examining bodies?
Is there:

- accreditation?
- supervised practice?
- an anatomy and physiology examination?
- a practical examination?
- a theory examination?
- support for the trainee therapist?

Does the course include business and communication skills?

Contact nurses who have been on the course, ask to visit the institution and talk to the teachers. If the organisation is reluctant to put you in touch with past pupils, or to receive personal visitors, that tells you something.

Cost is a significant factor for anyone considering going into complementary medicine. Successful practitioners certainly make a good living, and have the satisfaction of running their own business, but lucrative practices are not built up overnight and training can be long and expensive. Acupuncture, chiropractic, homeopathy and osteopathy, for example, involve three to four years' training, at a cost of £10,000-£15,000 or more. The costs of starting up a practice, and indemnity insurance, must also be considered.

**You are responsible**

Another factor to bear in mind is your likely working environment. Although many complementary practitioners work in groups, sharing premises and administrative staff, there is little teamwork of the type you experience in a hospital ward, operating theatre or general practice. You are likely to be working one to one nearly all the time with complete responsibility for diagnosis and treatment decisions. You need to be comfortable, and feel competent, with this sort of autonomy.

You should also think about the nature of the patient-practitioner relationship. Many complementary therapies involve considerable amounts of physical contact with patients and stress the importance of therapeutic touch. Will you be comfortable having this extensive physical contact with a huge variety of people, day after day?

## Acupuncture

Acupuncture is used to treat a wide range of problems including allergy, arthritis, asthma, back pain, headache, migraine, stress, ulcers, dermatitis, hypertension and depression. It involves the insertion of very fine needles at specified points, along lines of energy known as meridians. The acupuncture points are believed to be linked to internal organs. The needles are believed to unblock and increase or decrease the flow of energy through the meridians, and thus help maintain balance within the body.

Training is a three year or four year course leading to a Diploma or Licentiate in Acupuncture. Entrance requirements are generally two A levels, but Colleges are willing to consider other qualifications. Costs are up to £3,250 a year. Acupuncturists charge about £30 for an initial one hour consultation, less for subsequent visits.

## Aromatherapy

Aromatherapy involves using plant oils, usually in massage, to treat the mind and body. It is often combined with reflexology. The oils used are obtained from various parts of the plant including roots, stems, leaves and flowers and are highly concentrated. Aromatherapists maintain that

***Caroline Stevensen, aged 36,** is a sister in the Intensive Therapy Unit at the Middlesex Hospital, London, where she uses and teaches aromatherapy and shiatsu massage. She also runs a private practice in aromatherapy and shiatsu. She is a member of the steering committee of the RCN's Complementary Therapies in Nursing Special Interest Group and has carried out research into the benefits of massage for patients following heart surgery.*

**“Treating patients with complementary therapies gives me real satisfaction and a feeling of providing quality care. You feel that you have contributed to their wellbeing at a deeper level than you do simply with orthodox nursing. The tactile element, being able to reassure with touch as well as words, is enormously important. I think the main benefits of complementary therapies are psychological – they relieve anxiety, promote relaxation and help people to sleep.**

**I certainly see an increase in interest among nurses and doctors and I am called in where there are problems of intractable pain, or headaches, and I find that very satisfying. Doctors will consider complementary therapies as an option on the ward round now. At the moment I see private patients at home on my days off and the weekends. They come through word of mouth. I thought of going into private practice full time but I am more interested in integrating orthodox and complementary medicine.”**

essential oils can treat and relieve a variety of problems including asthma, constipation, depression, migraine, insomnia, poor circulation and fluid retention. The oils can be inhaled and used in baths or compresses as well as massage. Therapists use about 30 oils to treat most conditions.

The Aromatherapy Organisations Council recommends

that training should include 180 hours study (80 hours aromatherapy, 60 hours massage and 40 hours anatomy and physiology) and take a minimum of 9 months to complete. Aromatherapy is increasingly being used with elderly and cancer patients, and attracting growing interest from nurses. Aromatherapists in private practice charge £12-£30 for sessions lasting an hour and a half.

## Chiropractic

Chiropractic is used to treat acute and chronic pain, sports injuries and whiplash injuries. Most of the work is with musculo-skeletal problems such as low back pain and neck pain. The therapy includes manipulation and rotation of different parts of the spine to help muscle relaxation and restore normal movement to joints.

Training, at the Anglo-European College of Chiropractic, Bournemouth, is a four year full-time course leading to a BSc in Chiropractic. The course covers anatomy, physiology, biochemistry, therapeutics, radiology and chiropractic technique. Entrance requirements are generally three A levels, including chemistry and another science subject, but other qualifications will be considered. RGNs may be accepted on the proviso that they take extra tuition in chemistry first. The fees are £5,100 a year. Some local authority grants are available towards part of the cost.

There are some 500 chiropractors working in the UK. They charge between £15 and £35 per session. The first session is likely to last half and hour, with subsequent treatments of 15 minutes.

## Herbal medicine

Medical herbalism or phytotherapy has a long tradition dating back to ancient Egypt. Herbalists believe herbalism can be used to treat most conditions including arthritis, migraine and skin disorders. The treatment prescribed can be taken either as a tincture, infusion, compress, poultice, cream or ointment.

There are some 300 medical herbalists working in the UK in private practice. A four year full-time course is offered by the School of Phytotherapy (Herbal Medicine), leading to a Diploma in Phytotherapy, which makes the holder eligible for membership of the National Institute of Medical Herbalists. Entrance requirements are generally A levels in Biology and Chemistry but the School will consider relevant professional qualifications. Fees are more than £3,000 a year. The course covers biochemistry, philosophy, botany, clinical diagnosis, pharmacology, pathology and physiology.

The School of Phytotherapy also runs a four year correspondence course, leading to a Certificate in Phytotherapy. The course involves 30-40 hours study a week and 500 hours under clinical supervision in a clinic.

Medical herbalists charge around £16-20 for the first one hour consultation and about £10 for subsequent half-hour visits. There are some 200 working in the UK.

# Homeopathy

Homeopathy is based on the theory that substances which cause symptoms similar to those of a disease can stimulate the body to fight against that disease. Homeopathic remedies are made from plant, animal and mineral substances. The more diluted the solution the greater its potency.

Homeopathy stresses the uniqueness of the individual and remedies are prescribed for the whole person not the disorder. Homeopaths take into account patients' preferences, moods, emotions and how they speak and move, and their reactions to different sounds. The same symptom may be treated differently in different people.

There are some 15 colleges in the UK offering three year courses in homeopathy leading to a wide variety of qualifications. Entry requirements are generally two A levels but some colleges accept mature students with other qualifications. Homeopaths charge £20 to £50 for an initial consultation lasting one hour.

## Therapeutic massage

Therapeutic massage aims to relax and invigorate the mind and body. It is used in a wide variety of contexts, including cancer care and the rehabilitation of cardiac patients, to promote a sense of wellbeing and confidence. It is also used for sports injuries, during pregnancy, and for mothers and babies immediately after birth. It aims to improve the circulation, muscular and nervous systems.

An entire body massage takes 60-90 minutes. Four main types of movement are used: slow rhythmic strokes (effleurage), short fast movements (percussion), grasping and squeezing actions (petrissage) and friction. Practitioners work in offices and visit people's homes, as well as working in GPs' surgeries and private practice.

Many courses are available, most lasting between three and nine months, part time.

The London College of Massage offers a beginners' course involving a three hour session (day or evening) once a week for ten weeks, with one full day, or one weekend per month for three months.

The more advanced Practitioner Certificate course involves one three hour session a week for 12 weeks, plus homework treatments, case histories and practice classes. The College also offers an Advanced Practitioner Certificate course. Introductory weekends are also available. Fees start from £270 for the beginners' course.

The Northern Institute of Massage, Blackpool, offers a 12-15 month home study course, with a minimum of seven two-day practical sessions, in Blackpool or London, leading to a Diploma in Remedial Massage. The fee is £840.

# Osteopathy

There are some 2,000 osteopaths practising in the UK. *Which?* surveys published in 1986 and 1992 showed this was the most popular complementary therapy. Osteopathy is a system of diagnosis and treatment which emphasises the structural and mechanical problems of the body. The therapy involves manipulation, massage, stretching and thrusting techniques.

Most of the osteopath's work is concerned with spinal problems such as low back ache and neck pain, but osteopathy is also used to treat headaches, osteoarthritis, sports and dancing injuries. Osteopathic treatment is preceded by a detailed physical examination to assess the range and quality of movement in particular joints, and the state of muscles and ligaments.

The General Council and Register of Osteopaths accredits four year, full-time training courses at four schools. These include the British School of Osteopathy where the course leads to a BSc in Osteopathy. The fees are £5,800 a year.

Entrance requirements are generally two science A levels but equivalent experience will be considered. Osteopaths charge £15-£35 per consultation. The first consultation usually lasts 45 minutes; subsequent treatments 30 minutes.

# Reflexology

Reflexology, or zone therapy as it is sometimes known, is based on the belief that zones on the feet mirror different parts of the body. Practitioners maintain that by applying special massage techniques to the correct points of the foot they can can treat almost any organ or area of the body. It is believed that the left foot represents the left-hand side of the body and the right foot the right-hand side.

Different parts of the sole of the foot are thought to

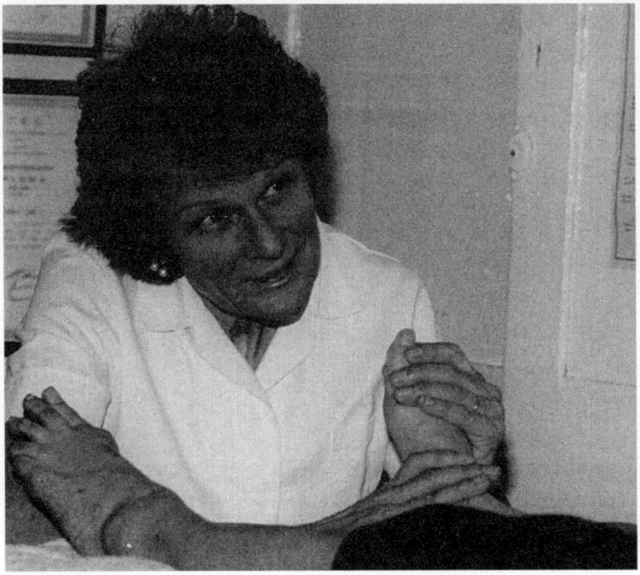

***Liz Gale**, aged 54, went into nursing at the age of 37, completing RGN training on a course for mature students at Queen Alexandra Hospital, Portsmouth. She has worked at Countess Mountbatten House, an NHS hospice in Southampton, and now runs her own complementary therapy practice giving massage, aromatherapy and reflexology. She also teaches hospice staff complementary therapies. She has a qualification in massage from the International Therapy Examination Council and a certificate in reflexology from the West London College of Reflexology.*

**“ I enjoy the hands-on aspect of complementary therapies and find it very satisfying to work one to one, and to be able to give people time. I also like the autonomy I have now. It is a fantastic feeling to watch someone unwind and relax under your hands. You can see the treatment making a difference.**

**I started by distributing 40 leaflets to people I knew**

**and the clients have all come through word of mouth. I think it is important to build up slowly and not take on more than you can handle. When someone has a medical problem, like a bad back, I always ask them to check with their doctor first before starting treatment.**

**You have to like people and be quite sensitive. Some people want to talk all the time during a treatment, others just want to relax. You need to go carefully with each person and put them at their ease. I think being a nurse certainly helps and makes people feel more relaxed. I never tell people that I can cure them, only that I think I can help them.**

**I would like to see complementary therapies widely used in the NHS because I think touching is so helpful. And communication becomes so much easier if you are doing something physical, like a hand massage. The number of people who come into hospital who have not been touched for years is frightening. ”**

connect in some way to such organs as the bladder, kidney and lungs, and the massage is believed to unblock energy channels in the body. Practitioners examine the soles, sides and tops of the feet, feeling for areas of tenderness. If one is found, the corresponding part of the body is thought to be out of balance. Neck pain, for example, is treated by applying pressure to the points at the base of the big toes. Reflexology is also used to treat back pain, headaches, tension and period pains.

Many part-time courses are available, generally lasting between two and nine months. Course fees vary from £150-£700. Practitioners charge £12-£25 per one hour session.

The International Therapy Examination Council, established in 1973, sets exams in many complementary therapies, leading to diploma and certificate qualifications. Many training centres offer courses based on its syllabus.

# 8 OPPORTUNITIES TO TRAVEL

• Half the group wish to go 'skinny-dipping' while the others are clearly embarrassed. What do you do/say?

• On leaving the hotel in the Dordogne with a group the proprietors give you a 500g tin of pate de foie gras. Do you accept or refuse?

• The private lives and scandals of British royalty arise in general conversation with the group. Do you:

- join in and try to stimulate conversation?
- join in but make only a non-committal contribution?
- say nothing?
- try to steer the conversation on to another topic?

*These are among the questions posed to prospective employees by one specialist travel company.*

Working in travel requires resourcefulness, stamina, tact and diplomacy. You must be able to think on your feet and be at ease coping with constant demands. Being very sociable and practical are prerequisites for success.

Thomson, Britain's largest tour operator, which employs some 2,000 staff overseas, asks applicants if they play a musical instrument and whether they have any experience in entertainment. Most travel companies expect a clean driving licence and proficiency in at least one European language besides English. The preferred age range for representatives is generally 21-35, and some specify that applicants should be single. Chalet reps are expected to ski and cook well.

You will be expected to satisfy clients' expectations, or at

***Fi Lowry**, aged 39, did a degree in Modern History and French at Edinburgh University before undertaking a two year SRN course at St Thomas's Hospital, London, followed by midwifery training. She has worked as a midwife in Abu Dhabi, in cardiac care in Baghdad and two years in acute medicine in Muscat. She also spent some time working for the National Trust in Scotland, sheep shearing on Fair Isle.*

*Now based in Italy, she speaks French and Italian and has been a tour leader for the Alternative Travel Group, which specialises in walking and trekking, since 1990. She is self-employed and leads tours in Tuscany, Umbria, the Dolomites and Sicily.*

**“ Being a good tour leader means sussing out each person's idea of a dream holiday and making sure they get it. If someone's particular interest is church music, for example, you must find a good concert and get them there. It's not unlike midwifery when you must find out about the individual's expectations and make sure their experience is as near to that as possible. But it's extremely hard work – 24 hours a day when you are on a trip – and you are required to respond on so many fronts all the time.**

**A sense of humour is vital. And you need to be sociable and able to get on with people at all levels and gain their confidence. We walk with the clients all day and always eat with them at night. It is important to be very enthusiastic and know about the area you are in, its food, wine, architecture and countryside.**

**The group dynamics can be quite difficult but nursing training helps there, too. You must recognise trouble and deal with it quickly. Some people arrive very wound up from their jobs. It helps to be able to keep a professional detachment. Being a nurse certainly boosts your credibility with clients and helps them relax. And I don't worry about clients getting ill. ”**

least minimise any disappointment, and remain accountable for everything you do to your employers back home. Many companies now issue clients with evaluation questionnaires at the end of each holiday, and your performance will be monitored all the time.

Hours are long and fairly irregular. You may be moved from town to town, or even country to country, during the season, according to the company's needs.

**On duty 24 hours a day**

The work varies from company to company, but travel reps with the large operators are expected to meet guests at the airport and transfer them by coach to their hotel, hold some form of welcome reception, arrange excursions and sort out any problems while they are there. On a walking or trekking holiday you may be expected to take part in all the daytime activity, as well as being responsible for overseeing hotel and meal arrangements. On a touring holiday you may also be responsible for transporting the luggage between hotels. You will be required to keep detailed records and report back to your employer.

Chalet reps are expected to shop and cook for the group each night, clean the rooms and be able to ski. Ski Guides are required to ski to an advanced level and may be responsible for organising evening entertainment. Working as a children's rep involves organising walks, beach games and treasure hunts, supervising meals and operating a patrolling service in the evenings.

Working in travel offers variety, an opportunity to live in a good climate with people who have come to enjoy themselves, and the chance to experience different cultures. You are likely to meet huge numbers of people and come into contact with many nationalities.

Although it is very unlikely to be restful, working as a rep, tour leader or tour manager can be a welcome break between permanent jobs, and give you time to consider your next move, in pleasant surroundings. Alternatively, you may find the way of life so congenial that you decide to make this your main occupation. Some tour leaders are self-employed and this provides flexibility to decide when, and how much, you will work.

Working in travel also provides opportunities to develop special interests such as sailing, bird-watching, trekking, painting and wild life. The number of specialist travel companies has grown considerably in the last ten years and it is worth considering working with one which matches your own interests. The Independent Guide to Real Holidays Abroad is a good source of addresses.

If you are proficient in a sport and think you would enjoy teaching it, you should consider applying to one of the holiday companies as an instructor.

Jobs as couriers and representatives are advertised in the Daily Express, Evening Standard, Daily Mail and Travel Trade Gazette. Most companies provide free accommodation, although this sometimes means sharing a room, and half or full board. Some offer travel concessions on completion of a specified period of service.

The work is usually seasonal: April to October for summer holidays and December to April for the ski season.

**Pay:** Variable. Some companies pay £250 a month into a UK bank account, plus cost of living allowance abroad. Self-employed reps can earn between £10 and £85 per day. Some companies offer commission on excursion sales.

# In-flight nursing

There are some 200 in-flight nurses in the UK and they are mainly self-employed working on contracts with medical assistance companies responsible for repatriating people who become ill abroad.

The job involves flying overseas, often at short notice, assessing the patient and his or her fitness to travel, all

***Richard Hough**, aged 33, RGN and RSCN, trained at the Westminster Hospital, and has held several posts in in medicine, surgery and accident and emergency. He has been working as a self-employed in-flight nurse since 1989, and is chair of the RCN's In-Flight Nurses Special Interest Group.*

**“ I went into in-flight nursing because I wanted some independence and autonomy, and more direct patient contact. I like the variety and challenge. The work involves repatriating sick people from abroad, both on scheduled airlines and private planes. You need to be resourceful – getting telephone lines out of Greek islands can be difficult – willing to take responsiblity and able to make decisions on your own.**

**You must assess the sick person's fitness to travel, make arrangements for getting them on to the plane, take complete responsibility for their care during the flight, and accompany them to hospital on arrival in the UK. With a seriously ill patient you are running a sort of mini intensive care unit at the back of the plane. You have to be agile and able to transport equipment.**

**In exceptional cases you have to decide whether to ask the captain to make an unscheduled landing, involving huge extra costs and disruption to other passengers.**

**We spend about 15 hours with the patient on average, but it can be longer if you have to stay with them until they are well enough to fly. And repatriating someone from Australia means working for 36 hours at a stretch. You get to know people intensely for a short period.**

**It is important to be able to establish a rapport with the sick person and any relatives very quickly, and to give them confidence. The relatives may have been left alone in a strange hotel wondering what is going to happen and can be extremely stressed. You may the first person who has spoken English to them for a week. But**

**they are usually delighted to see us and extremely grateful to come home.**

**You need to be flexible and able to deal with cabin crew, ground staff and local hospitals and have enough of the local language to slow down an ambulance as you are tearing through the countryside!**

**The work is seasonal, and somewhat unpredictable, but very gratifying. And varied, certainly. I was part of the Virgin Atlantic medical team that went to Baghdad in October 1990 to bring back the 35 hostages who were released on medical grounds, before the Gulf War. You must always be prepared to take off at short notice. I keep £300-£400 in 16 different currencies. ”**

nursing care during the flight and accompanying the person to hospital on arrival in the UK.

Assignments can range from sick babies, to adolescents injured in scooter accidents on the Greek Islands, and elderly stroke patients. The majority of patients are over 70.

The job requires an ability to work on your own, resourcefulness (you will have to deal with ground crew of varying helpfulness and local hospital staff) and a manner which inspires confidence.

The stress of illness and accident are intensified away from home. An important part of the in-flight nurse's role is to bring swift reassurance to both patient and relatives, who may be distraught and completely disorientated by what has happened, and unable to speak the local language. You must be able to build up a relationship quickly, as on most trips you will spend little more than a day with your patient.

Physical fitness is also required. You may have to set up the equivalent of a small intensive care unit at the back of the plane, and manoeuvre a stretcher on and off the aircraft, with little space in which to turn around. On some occasions you may be called on to provide assistance if one of the other passengers becomes ill.

**A high degree of responsibility**

This is a very specialised form of nursing which is not for everybody. It suits those who are adaptable, self-reliant and happy to take a high degree of responsibility. But it does not offer the chance of following up patients and caring for them until recovery. The work certainly offers travel but few trips include time for looking around. Work is seasonal with the most intense demand during the summer months.

Companies usually require several years experience in accident and emergency and intensive care. Reputable companies interview applicants and follow up references. Living near a major airport is an advantage as many trips start very early in the morning.

**Pay:** £18,000-£21,000 pro rata.

**Training:** A 12-day In-Flight Nursing course is offered by the Institute of Advanced Nursing Studies.

# Immunisation clinics

There are some three dozen travel immunisation clinics in the UK. These are run by British Airways Medical Services for Travellers Abroad (BAMSTA) with several operated on a franchise basis. The clinics maintain a database of the immunisation requirements of every country in the world. The larger clinics provide up to 2,500 vaccinations a month, and most run appointments systems.

The work is generally nine to five but there are some part-time and job sharing opportunities. Training is provided. The work requires good interpersonal skills, a taste for meeting large numbers of the public, and some interest in sales work. The clinics sell products such as anti-malaria tablets, water purifiers and filters and mosquito repellants.

**Pay:** £15,000-£17,500

**Holidays:** 4-6 weeks

# Nursing on a cruise ship

Working on a cruise ship offers the chance to see the world, travel in comfortable circumstances and enjoy a good social life. It can be very satisfying if you are sociable, outgoing, good at working in a small team and at ease in the world of private medicine.

Cruise ships are a world apart, dedicated to enjoyment, and offer the chance to observe human behaviour and emotions under very special circumstances. They also provide their share of medical emergencies as well as the routine work of seasickness, coughs and strains. Part of the work involves running a small ward. You will be responsible

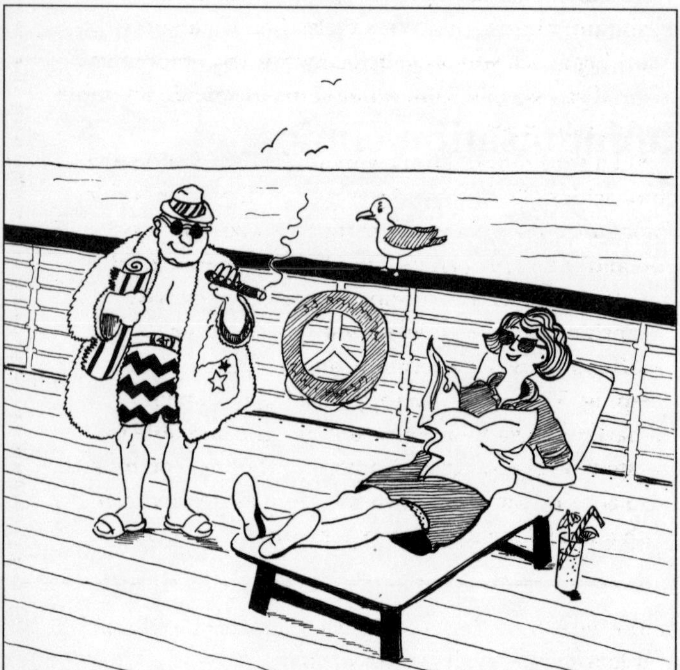

Eve Morris

*The chance to see the world, travel in comfortable circumstances and enjoy a good social life...*

*__Denise Donnelly__, aged 45, trained in Liverpool, qualified as a midwife, and has worked in France, Canada and the Far East. She also spent five years working on P&O cruise liners, where she was responsible, with two other nurses and a doctor, for the health of 2,000 passengers and crew. She is now a community nurse in London.*

**“I loved the life at sea. It was very hard work – we had to provide a 24-hour service – but varied and quite glamorous. You could be eating in the restaurant one minute and dealing with a cardiac arrest the next. We held two surgeries a day and ran a ward of 15 beds. We also carried out immunisation programmes for the crew.**

**The most common problems were seasickness and respiratory infections, but we also had accidents. Working at sea you must be ready for any emergency, from distress calls from other ships to suicide attempts and bomb scares.**

**On a four month cruise you might have ten deaths, and visiting the bereaved was part of the nurse's role. Relationships can also seem much more emotional at sea and the nurse can be called on to listen and advise on affairs, excessive promiscuity and pregnancy.**

**Working at sea requires a sense of humour, confidentiality, co-operation and excellent record keeping. You must be happy working in a small department yet be interested in people and able to relate to everyone from Captain to Rating. You must also accept that you are working in private medicine, with all the demands and expectations that involves.”**

for the health of the crew, as well as passengers, and must be able to relate to all groups of staff.

As a lot of the passengers are elderly, and deaths not infrequent, you may also find yourself in a counselling role, supporting the bereaved. You may also have to support crew members who are concerned about problems back home.

The work requires tact, a sense of humour, and an understanding that life at sea gives a special perspective. Emotions are often heightened and some passengers find taking a relaxing break from problems back home is not as easy as they thought. Some may find the enclosed world of a ship difficult to adjust to.

Patients will expect a lot of attention, and sensitivity is required. On board ship you never get away from work and will be expected to mix with passengers at night. A high proportion of passengers are likely to be American, which means you must keep meticulous records in case of malpractice suits.

Companies recruit RGNs with several years experience, preferably in accident and emergency, intensive care and private medicine. Overseas nursing experience, particularly in the Middle East, is also an advantage. Some companies also require applicants to be registered midwives.

Applicants must be fit and the preferred age is 25-35. Some companies offer full-time employment and others employ nurses on contracts of a few months.

**Pay:** Around or below NHS rates.

# 9 OVERSEAS OPPORTUNITIES

A national study of 4,000 nurses in the UK, published by the Institute of Manpower Studies and the RCN in September 1992, showed one in five was considering working abroad, and ten per cent of qualified nurses had held a nursing job outside the UK. The most popular destinations were Australia, Canada and the USA, Saudi Arabia having dropped in appeal following the Gulf War. There was little movement of UK nurses to work in other European Community countries.

Some 8,000 qualified nurses left the UK in 1990/91 with the intention of working abroad. The research also showed that about half those considering working abroad were under 30 and single. The average length of stay abroad was relatively short – two years or less.

**Stepping off the career ladder?**

The study also found that nurses who had worked abroad were more likely to remain outside the NHS on their return, working for agencies or the independent sector. Anecdotal evidence suggests that overseas experience is not always viewed positively by the NHS and nurses returning from abroad may have to accept a lower grade than they were previously working at.

A spell overseas will broaden your outlook, increase your confidence, and give you a new perspective on health, culture and politics. It may also offer a chance to improve your bank balance. But it may not automatically provide a step up the career ladder back home, and this is certainly a factor to bear in mind when considering working abroad.

**International Office of the RCN**

Anyone considering nursing work abroad should contact the International Office of the RCN. It accepts telephone inquiries from non-members and has a wide range of

*__Mhairi Allan,__ aged 33, did her RGN training in Glasgow, and worked in The Armed Forces Hospital in Oman from 1985 to 1988. Her overseas experience also includes three months as a volunteer on Operation Raleigh in Australia, two years as an intensive care nurse on Grand Cayman in the West Indies and three months in Saudi Arabia. She is now doing agency work and studying for a degree in dance.*

**“I went abroad for a better lifestyle, as well as to broaden my experience, and the conditions in Oman were excellent. I made £1,500 a month tax free, and had free accommodation – a two bedroom house with a swimming pool – car and petrol. It was very sociable and there were lots of sports. The hospital had just opened; it was very well equipped and the staff/patient ratios were good. But there was no ambulance service and the injuries were worse than those you see in the UK – a lot of head injuries and traffic accidents.**

**On Operation Raleigh I was responsible, with one doctor, for 50 volunteers in several camps spread throughout Victoria. We had to teach first aid and monitor the sanitary conditions. There were a lot of stomach upsets, and sprains and some minor burns. There was radio contact between the camps but you had to be very resourceful and anticipate problems. I found it quite stressful.**

**In Grand Cayman I was working as staff nurse in a small general hospital which was extremely hard work.**

**You need to be adaptable and self-reliant to work abroad, but the experience develops confidence and makes you less scared about change.”**

written material for members. This includes general information on working abroad and the opportunities available, guidance on earnings, taxation and national insurance, professional indemnity insurance, provision for medical treatment, recognition of professional courses undertaken abroad, and re-entry.

The International Office provides a contract checklist with information on employment conditions. It can supply up-to-date guidance on the nursing scene, and registration requirements in various countries, including Australia, Canada, the USA and New Zealand. The Office also maintains a list of social contacts around the world.

The RCN guidance stresses the importance of checking overseas contracts thoroughly, in writing, before signing, as there is unlikely to be much room for negotiation afterwards. Points to check include:

**Salaries**

- Is the salary fixed or is it on an hourly rate? If it is an hourly rate this could mean that if there is not a sufficient number of patients to treat you will not be required to work and therefore will not be paid.
- If the salary is on a scale, at what level have you been offered employment?
- Is the salary adequate for your needs? Check the cost of living with the relevant embassy.
- Where will the salary be paid? UK, host country or both?
- Is there a clause in the contract to safeguard you against possible falls in the exchange rate of the pound sterling?

**Hours**

- Make sure your hours of work are written into your contract. In some countries you may be expected to work longer than a 37-hour week. This can be very tiring in a different climate and in a new job.

**Shift work**

- Establish whether employment is for a specified shift such as night duty only. There may be no chance of transferring.

**Overtime**

- Will you be expected to do overtime regularly?
- Will it be necessary for you to do overtime to maintain an adequate standard of living?
- What rate will be paid for any overtime?

**Length of contract**

- Check the length of contract offered and on what terms it is renewable. A one-year contract may be best if you do not know the country, or have not worked abroad before.

**Annual leave**

- Is the annual leave adequate for your needs, bearing in mind that you will be working in another country and possibly for longer hours?
- Can you take your annual leave during the year or do you have to complete a year's contract first?
- Will the company pay your return air fare to the UK for your annual leave?

**Emergency and compassionate leave**

- Under what circumstances will this be granted?

**Accommodation**

- Is accommodation provided with the job?
- What is the cost?
- Is it single, or will it involve sharing?
- Who pays for gas, electricity, water, sewerage, telephone?
- If the employer does not provide accommodation, do they provide assistance in finding somewhere to live?

**Transport**

- Is local transport available to get you between your accommodation and the hospital? Who pays for this?
- If you are going to the USA, will you have enough money to buy a car on arrival? Many private American hospitals are in rural areas where public transport is non-existent.

**Medical and dental insurance**

- Is the employer providing insurance and is it adequate to cover private medical costs in the host country? What are

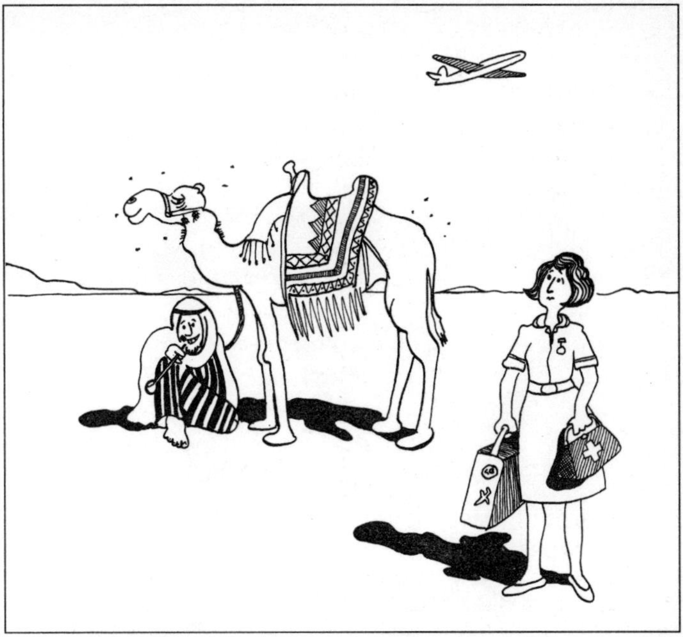

Eve Morris

*Is local transport available to get you to the hospital?*

the provisions for being flown home if you become ill, and who decides whether or not this is necessary?

**Sickness payments**

- Will all or only part of your salary be paid? For how long?

**Job description and nursing responsibilities**

- Is there a job description and are you satisfed with it? Are you being employed for specific nursing duties in a named specialty of nursing?

The contract probably gives your employer the right to alter your job description without consulting you.

It is very important to have complete understanding between you and the employer about the exact nature of your duties before you sign the contract. Nursing duties vary from country to country and you may be expected to undertake some tasks considered the province of medical or technical staff in the UK. Nurses should be certain that they are trained to undertake these procedures and are competent and happy to do so.

**Termination of the contract**

• How much notice do you have to give the employer before you can terminate the contract? What notice does the employer have to give you?

• Is there a penalty clause if you break the contract before its expiry date?

• If you are dismissed do you have to reimburse the outward air fare? Will your fare home be paid?

• Is there a bonus on successful completion of the contrct?

The RCN also advises that the prospective employee should be supplied with copies of any documents referred to in the contract, such as job description, local labour laws and benefits booklets.

# Working in the Middle East

Nursing in the Middle East provides opportunities to work with multi-national teams in well-equipped hospitals, experience Muslim culture, save some money and live in free accommodation. Salaries are not as high, relative to the UK, as they were in the 1980s, and recruiting organisations report fewer openings and lower turnover. Nurses already out there are tending to stay longer, possibly as a result of cuts and employment difficulties in the UK. But there are openings, particularly for midwives and those experienced in intensive care, renal dialysis and neonatology.

The jobs require physical fitness, stamina (the working week tends to be longer than the UK) flexibility, a sense of humour and considerable powers to adapt.

Work is offered on single status contracts, and applicants must be ready to accept the restrictions of living in a Muslim country. Women are not allowed to drive in Saudi

Arabia, alcohol is forbidden, and mixed bathing is prohibited in public places. Many hospitals, however, have social clubs and sports centres for staff, with opportunities for swimming, squash, tennis and badminton. Several of the hospitals are near the sea, providing opportunities for scuba diving. Nurses report a lively social life among the expatriate community, including amateur dramatics.

Most companies require nurses to have several years' post-registration experience, and some will not consider applicants under 25. Some locum posts are available.

A bonus of 15 days' salary is generally paid for every year of service completed, and some companies offer a return ticket to the UK every six months. The salaries are tax free.

**Pay - Saudi Arabia**
SEN, 44 hour week – £10,800-£12,000
RGN, 44 hour week – £14,400-£18,000
Junior sister, 44 hour week – £19,200
Senior Sister 44 hour week – £21,600
Director of Nursing – £50,000

SEN, 48 hour week – £12,500
RGN, 48 hour week – £15,500

**Holidays:** Variable but 49 days is usual.

# Working in a developing country

Working in a developing country means dropping your preconceptions and established ways of practising and adapting your experience to the needs and resources of the local population.

Part of your role will be to pass on your knowledge to the local health workers and help them develop their own health services. Agencies sending Western staff to developing countries encourage them to look on their relationship with local people as one of partnership rather than teacher/pupil.

Your clinical experience, particularly in areas such as midwifery, will almost certainly be broadened beyond what is available in the UK, and working without the back-up of well equipped hospitals is likely to increase your self-reliance, and confidence in your own skills.

You need to be adaptable, willing to learn, and able to integrate yourself into a foreign, and often remote, community for an extended period, with little or no contact with other expatriates. Most of the contracts offered by organisations such as Voluntary Service Overseas are for two years. You are likely to be paid the local rate for the job, plus all your travelling and removal expenses. Some organisations pay a monthly allowance in the UK.

Agencies sending nurses to work in developing countries usually require at least two years post-registration experience. Applicants who have already worked in a developing country are at an advantage. Midwifery and paediatric experience are particularly valuable. The average age of workers sent by one agency is 35.

**International Health Exchange**

Formerly the Bureau for Overseas Medical Service, the International Health Exchange maintains a register of health posts available in developing countries through some 40 organisations including VSO, Save the Children and the Catholic Institute for International Relations. It also produces a newsletter and provides training courses, including one on Primary Health Care in Developing Countries. It maintains an emergency register of health workers available for disaster relief work. The registration fee is £12-£35 according to your personal circumstances.

**NHS Overseas Enterprises**

Describing itself as the international marketing arm of the NHS, NHSOE was set up in 1988 to export UK health expertise and management skills and generate income for the NHS. Senior managers and tutors from the NHS are sent on secondment to overseas countries to help develop local health services and set up training programmes. The UK employee's salary, and a daily allowance, are paid by the client country and the individual returns to his/her NHS job at the end of the secondment. The arrangement offers NHS staff a chance to broaden their experience with a period abroad, without having to give up their job.

NHSOE offers expertise in a range of areas including acute services, primary care, elderly care, hospital maintenance, health education and health finance. It has provided advisers to Bangladesh, Bahrain, Fiji, India, Kuwait, Malaysia, Oman, Pakistan, Philippines, Qatar, Saudi Arabia, Spain, Turkey, United Arab Emirates, Uganda and Zambia and is developing projects in Eastern Europe.

Nurse managers and those with experience in nurse education interested in taking part should supply NHSOE with an up-to-date curriculum vitae, and some indication of the length of time, type of project and part of the world they would like to work in. Details will be recorded on database and considered when future projects come up.

## Summer work in the USA

BUNACAMP offers RGNs posts as infirmary assistants working in summer camps for children and young people under the guidance of US doctors and nurses. You get a return flight, food and accommodation and 560 dollars on completion of nine weeks work. The season runs from June to the middle or end of August and you will work a shift system, with one day off a week. BUNACAMP advertisements offer "a rewarding and challenging summer" for those who "like the outdoor life, don't mind hard work and have a genuine interest in working with children."

# 10 WORKING FOR A CHARITY / RUNNING A HELPLINE

The last ten years have seen the establishment of several new charities which offer telephone information lines staffed by nurses, such as BACUP (British Association of Cancer United Patients), CancerLink and the Medical Advisory Service, a small charity set up by two nurses in 1986 to give advice on all aspects of health care. Older charities such as the British Diabetic Association, the British Heart Foundation, the Multiple Sclerosis Society and the National Asthma Campaign also employ nurses.

Working for a charity requires flexibility, the ability to get on with a wide range of people, organisational and writing skills (as someone with a nursing background you will almost certainly be asked to help with information leaflets and publications) and diplomacy.

A taste for research and interpretation also help, as part of your job may be producing fact sheets and summarising clinical information for general readers.

Charities offer fairly regular hours, opportunities for part-time work and, in many cases, the chance to build up expertise in a specialist area. But you are likely to be working in an office environment, and the jobs are unlikely to suit those who derive most satisfaction from the bustle of a busy ward and hands-on nursing.

Many of your contacts will be on the telephone, or by letter, and there will often be no follow up. Working on a telephone helpline requires special communication skills, including the ability to deal with the unpredictable, and some find it draining, at least initially. The work can be intense, coping with high levels of distress from callers.

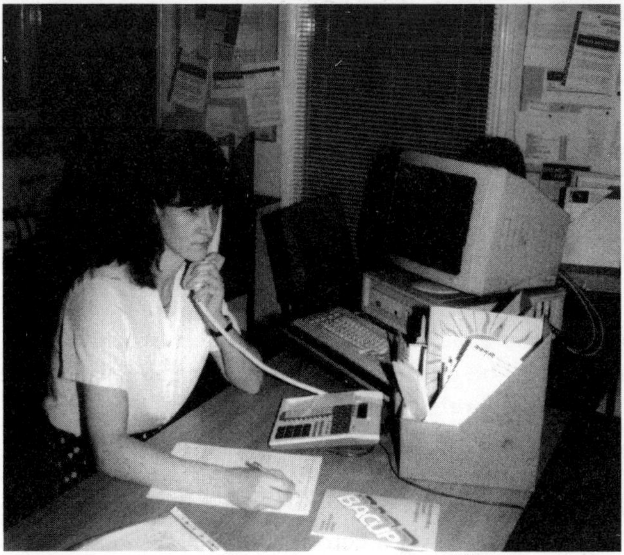

***Debbie Coats, aged 29,*** *trained at Walsgrave Hospital, Coventry, and has worked at Charing Cross Hospital and the Royal Marsden Hospital, Fulham, where she gained her Oncology Nursing Certificate. She joined BACUP, the British Association of Cancer-United Patients, in June 1991. The charity's helpline answers 140 calls a day.*

**“ Talking to people over the telephone is very different from having face-to-face contact with patients. But we get a lot of feedback which is very satisfying. The work is extremely varied and less stressful than working on a ward. There is time to read journals, go to conferences and keep up to date. When we are not on the telephone we do research and work on fact sheets. We have a good library and very good support from experts we can consult when we don't know something.**

**The range of calls is enormous: where to get insurance, emotional reactions to cancer, questions about death. About 70 per cent of calls are from**

**relatives or friends; people are often in great distress. That can be difficult but the nurses here give each other a lot of support; you don't feel you are working alone. And when you are on the telephone you can give the caller all the time they need. That's a real bonus. ”**

It is a mistake to look upon charities as calm havens. Most do not have the rigid hierarchy of a hospital but they have their share of office politics, and there may well be conflicts between the committee of volunteers who run the charity and the paid employees. In a small operation you may be faced with the idiosyncrasies of a founder who is reluctant to let go of any aspect of the organisation.

Find out as much as possible about the charity before applying for a job, both through word of mouth and your own research. Ask for a copy of the annual report and see what impression it gives of the organisation. Modern and professional? Developing and aware of changes in social policy? Or long established and low key? Are the medical advisers well known and respected in their field, or retired people you have never heard of? Look at the the figures and see how healthy the finances are – this could have a direct bearing on your job security.

The Charities Digest, published by Family Welfare Enterprises, 501-505 Kingsland Road, London E8 4AU, price £14.95, is a good starting point, giving the background and scope of over 700 charities. It is available in public libraries.

**Pay:** Several charities running helplines pay nurses on G grade: £16,200 - £18,750.

**Holidays:** 5-6 weeks

**Training:** Some but by no means all charities require specialist nursing qualifications in their clinical area. Many offer their own training in communication skills.

# 11 WORKING IN A RESIDENTIAL OR NURSING HOME

Working with elderly people in nursing homes and residential care homes requires sensitivity, compassion and commitment. The focus and pace are quite different from an acute setting. The work demands an empathy with elderly people and a determination to make each individual's life as comfortable and fulfilling as possible.

This is by no means easy and often requires subtlety and great patience both with clients, and their relatives. Good care requires that each person is treated as an individual, with respect for their independence, personality, tastes and habits. But it may be difficult to see the individual behind the disabling illness, which may have changed the personality and diminished or destroyed communication skills. In these circumstances it can be extremely difficult to build up a picture of the person's life, and personality, before they came into care, particularly if there are no relatives, and staff must rely on their own perceptions and experience.

**Feelings of loss**

The work also requires an appreciation of the complex emotions involved in a move to a residential or nursing home, for the family as well as the old person. The older person will almost certainly have a great sense of loss, for their previous way of life, identity and independence, combined with apprehension about the future, concern about their progressive dependence and fear of being abandoned by those close to them.

***Linda Nazarko,** aged 37, is matron of a 40-bed private nursing home in Croydon, Surrey, where she has worked for ten years. She trained at King's College Hospital, London, and has worked at the Maudsley Hospital, London and spent two years in Saudi Arabia.*

**“ There is a tremendous amount of scope working in nursing homes which are, after all, nurse-led units where the doctors only come by invitation. The quality of life is really up to the nurses.**

**And there is a lot you can do to improve things. We have reduced the incontinence rate from 54 per cent to 14 per cent with a continence programme, for example. And the introduction of a healthy, high-fibre diet has meant we only have one person on laxatives.**

**We have monthly patient meetings so that residents can let us know what their priorities are.**

**Working in a nursing home requires an open mind, enthusiasm, respect for patients' autonomy and readiness to act as their advocates. You must be assertive to make sure they get what they need, whether it is a wheelchair, hearing aid or physiotherapy.**

**It is satisfying to see people improve with rehabilitation and it's also satisfying to assist patients to a peaceful death. It's very different from hospital nursing but you have the chance to get to know people.**

**Now we need to raise the profile of care of the elderly and build bridges between the private sector and the NHS. We must also ensure nurses receive part of their training in nursing homes. If an area of nursing is not good enough for students it is not good enough for patients.**

**There's a huge amount to be done. Elderly care is still a Cinderella service. But good homes can have a ripple effect to raise standards. ”**

The person may also feel resentment at going into a situation where, however homely the setting, they will be living with others they do not know, and might not choose to know under other circumstances.

Relatives, too, will have a sense of loss and may feel inadequate and sad if they have been caring for the person themselves and are no longer able to do so, for whatever reason. Many feel guilty in some way even if there is no reason for doing so.

This is not to say all this cannot be alleviated, and in some cases transformed, with good support from sensitive staff. In time the older person may settle in and the feeling of being cared for, and not having to worry about their own safety, or maintaining their own home, may compensate for any feeling of loss.

But it does need sustained commitment and good communication skills. Older people in care homes need a great deal of emotional support and their sense of security and ease is hugely dependent on staff attitudes, and how they are treated over day-to-day activities. To work effectively staff must have a respect for each individual's worth and value, irrespective of the person's capabilities and personal appeal, or otherwise.

**A sense of self-worth**

A good nurse can give the person a sense of self-worth with everything she or he does. A routine task carried out with care and cheerfulness while communicating with the resident, rather than in a rushed impersonal way, can make all the difference in the world.

This is true of all areas of nursing, but is particularly important in long term care, where the majority of those being looked after are physically vulnerable and unlikely to regain full independence. This is a very special kind of caring. It offers opportunities to build up long-term relationships with residents, and to make a real difference to the quality of their lives.

***Shirley Englebright, aged 57,** went into nursing at the age of 35, trained at the Queen Victoria Hospital, East Grinstead, Sussex, and then spent six years as a district nurse. In 1981 she set up Stildon, a 20-bed residential home for the elderly, in East Grinstead, run by a trust. She is manager of the home and vice-chairman of the RCN's Residential Care Managers group.*

**“ The average age of our residents is 90 and it's very challenging to make sure someone of that age has a good day. I started Stildon with the aim of making each person comfortable and happy, able to do as much as possible. We must help people to see what they still have, and can still do, rather than what they have lost.**

**This sort of work is not for everyone, especially if you want the drama of acute care. But it is satisfying to care for people for a long time, and you get much more closely involved. In hospital you may care for someone for weeks. But some of our residents have been here ten years. When people die there is a great sense of loss for us, but they die in a safe environment, where they are known. In this work individual tastes and choice are very important. I would certainly want my preferences and tastes to be known. I wouldn't appreciate a milky cup of tea, or sugar in my coffee, for example, if I had never had that before.**

**Offering people choice is essential if you want them to feel at home, and it does not create problems. Care for your staff is essential for a good home, and it is vital to build up relationships with the community outside. We have school pupils here on work experience and a Friends group which helps with fundraising. Good relationships with the local doctors are also important.**

**Of course moving into a home is a big adjustment and I always try to visit people in their own homes before they come. And I suggest they come for a fortnight first,**

**before making any decision or selling their home.**

**Working in a residential home requires patience, a sense of humour, tact, and kindness. The residents always say they need kindness more than anything else. You must also be able to listen and pick up the underlying messages.**

**I think things have improved in the last ten years and care of the elderly is increasingly seen as challenging and worthwhile. But there is still a long way to go. ”**

Local authority and NHS provision for old people has diminished in the last ten years and the majority of beds are now in private homes. These range from small husband and wife operations, looking after a dozen, or fewer, residents to large, purpose built homes, run by commercial operators and housing more than 100 residents or patients.

Standards of care vary enormously in long term care, and are not simply a reflection of the fees charged. Placement agencies advising health authorities and families on homes report that two homes in the same area can be charging more or less the same fees and yet differ dramatically in atmosphere and approach.

Bearing this in mind, anyone considering working in a particular home should find out as much as possible about it. What is its reputation locally? With local GPs and community nurses, and families? It is worthwhile trying to meet staff already working there to ask them about standards, conditions and atmosphere.

You should also be aware that in the private sector the onus is on you to negotiate acceptable terms and to clarify any points you are unsure about. Some small homes value their staff and treat them fairly but others seem chiefly concerned with keeping costs down. You may get a better employment package working for one of the large operators owning several homes.

Nursing and residential care homes offer good opportunities for part-time and shift work, and some jobs provide staff accommodation, such as a flat, but the rates of pay are often lower than the NHS.

**Pay :**

Home Director, 90-bed nursing home, Scotland
– £23,000 plus performance related pay (PRP)
Matron, private nursing home, South Coast – £17,000
RGNs, nursing home, Bedfordshire – £13,801-£16,801
RGN, nursing home, London – £13,760
Manager, care home, Warwickshire – £19,000 plus PRP
Deputy Manager, residential home, London – £17,074
Care assistants – £2.75 per hour

Hourly rates: RGNs – £5.00-£7.50
ENs – £4.43-£6.98
RGN in charge – £5.39-£8.00

Permanent posts are usually for 40 hours a week

**Holidays:** three to four weeks.

Some employers like nurses to have completed the English National Board's Nursing for Elderly People Course (ENB 941). This is a 22-day course, available on a day release basis, to be completed within six months.

**Starting your own care home**

Information on exactly what is involved in purchasing and setting up your own nursing or residential home can be obtained from the professional associations listed in the *Directory of Useful Contacts and Addresses* at the end of this book. You should also contact the homes registration officer at your local social services department or health authority.

# 12 WORKING AS A NANNY

PARIS – Famous French film director needs top nanny. Travel between fully staffed home in Paris and Normandy. Children 5 years, 3 years and 7 months. French useful for this highly sought-after position. £180 per week negotiable.

ITALY, near Turin – Maternity nurse required for triplets due late December. Three months assignment £300+ per week.

BUCKINGHAMSHIRE – Nanny required as soon as possible for sole charge of three adorable children. Driver, car provided, non-smoker, swimmer (own pool). Two bedroom flat, holidays skiing, Wales and France. Good pay and conditions.

LONDON W8 – Permanent part-time daily nanny required for every Thursday. Sole charge of beautiful bouncy boy, 3 months. 8am-7pm. £35-£40 per day.

*Advertisements from Nursery World.*

Working as nanny can be a happy and fulfilling experience, offering variety and a chance to sample life at different strata of society, and in different countries. It also offers a variety of work patterns: full time living-in, full time daily, part time, temporary and a variety of nanny sharing arrangements.

Nurses are popular as nannies, and particularly as maternity nurses, caring for newborn babies in their first weeks at home. If you are qualified as a Registered Sick Children's Nurse (RSCN) or in midwifery, you will be in a particularly strong position when looking for jobs.

But working as a nanny is quite different from working in a hospital, where the pattern of life is largely determined by the medical and nursing staff. Working in a family, whether it is that of a one-parent career woman in Islington, or

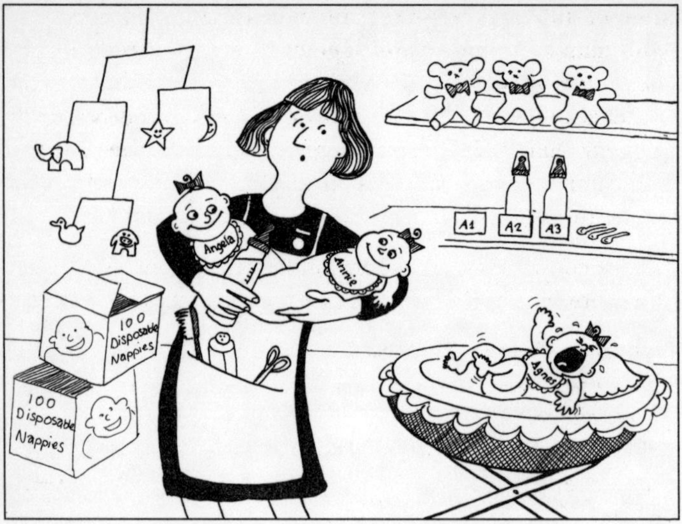


Eve Morris

*Will you have "sole charge" or share care with parents?*

several generations of gentry in their country seat, requires flexibility and adaptability, plus self-assurance, consistency, and confidence in your own values.

While your primary focus should be the physical and emotional needs of the child, or children, you must be able to fit into the family group, and endorse the parents' values and standards as far as possible. Obviously, the extent to which this is expected of you will vary from job to job and a temporary, daily nanny will not be expected to integrate as much as a permanent, resident one. But if you feel really out of sympathy with the set-up no arrangement will be very happy for either side. So it is extremely important to sort out the conditions in as much detail as possible before taking any job. This cannot be emphasised too strongly.

It is also important to bear in mind that a family can be one of the trickiest, and most emotionally demanding, work situations. While you may be made the friend and confidante of one or both parents you must try to remain calm and impartial in good times and bad. Being one of the family yet still an employee is not an easy balancing act.

Jobs, many through nanny agencies, are advertised in *The Lady*, *Nursery World* and *Nursing Times.* If you have not worked as a nanny before it is probably wise to register with an agency which will be able to give you an overview of the employment scene and what to expect. They could also save you time and help clarify what you are looking for.

Before contacting an agency it is worth summarising what you are hoping for:

- a post in a specific town/area?
- live in or daily?
- part-time or full-time?
- permanent or temporary?
- single new baby? twins? established family with several children?
- "sole charge" or sharing care with parent/s?

In permanent positions, in the UK and abroad, you will be expected to stay at least a year.

When you meet your prospective employer/s it is important to clarify the following points:

**Salary and method of payment**

What will you be paid and how? Weekly, monthly, cash, cheque, banker's order? It is the employer's duty to pay the nanny's tax and national insurance.

**Hours of work and holidays**

Agree on hours of work and days and weekends off.

**Living arrangements**

Ask to see your bedroom and the bathroom you will be expected to use. Will you be expected to share the bathroom with other members of the family or guests? Always or occasionally?

**Meals**

Where will meals be taken? Will you eat with the parents

***Marie Owens, aged 30,*** *trained as an SEN at St Helier hospital, Carshalton, Surrey, and then worked as an agency nurse and school matron. She started work as a nanny when she took a holiday job, looking after a two-year-old who had undergone major heart surgery and had a tracheostomy. She spent more than two years with the family and is now in her third nanny post, looking after triplets aged nine months, in London. She has a Montessori Nursery Teaching Diploma.*

**“ I like the closeness you have with children as a nanny, and seeing them develop. I only take jobs where I have sole charge and parents certainly find it reassuring to know I am a nurse. But you do find yourself having to diagnose every spot.**

**Being a nanny is a totally different ball game from nursing. You have to slow down and go at the child's pace. And you've got to be flexible and fit in to the parents' lifestyle. I think in some ways being a nanny is harder than nursing because once you are in a job you tend to live it, and work 12- hour days. And it can be difficult leaving. Leaving my first job was terrible.**

**It is vital to get everything sorted out at the beginning. Don't ever take a job without a contract and if you have any anxiety at all, discuss it before you start. ”**

occasionally, or all the time? If you are expected to cook for yourself in the evening who provides the food and where do you cook it?

**Duties**

Will you be expected to cook for the children? Look after their clothes? Clean their bedroom or playroom? Will you be expected to babysit and if so how often? If the baby wakes in the night who will be responsible for getting up? Will you be in "sole charge" of the baby, child or children, or does the mother expect to share looking after the children? On a regular basis? Just when she happens to be at home?

**Trial period and notice required**
What will these be?

**Car**
Will you be allowed the use of a car? Will you be expected to drive the children to school, playgroup, or parties? All the time or occasionally?

**Uniform**
Will you be expected to wear one?

**Smoking**
It is important to establish their attitude to smoking, if you are a smoker. Most families will ask you not to smoke near the children. But what about in your own room when you are off duty? Similarly, if you or the family are vegetarian, how will you cope with this? And what will the children eat? At home and when they are out?

If you have the opportunity to spend a day or two with the family before accepting the job, or to meet the previous nanny, do so.

**Contracts**
You and and your future employer should sign a contract. The Federation of Recruitment and Employment Services (FERES), the trade association for the private recruitment industry, supplies nanny agencies with model nanny contracts (available to individuals with SAE) for posts in the UK and overseas.

The contract covers pay, hours of work, pensions, sickness, insurance, discipline and termination. It also covers confidentiality: "It is a condition of employment that now and at all times in the future, save as may be lawfully required, the employee shall keep the affairs and concerns of the household and its transactions and business confidential". It outlines the procedure to be followed in the case of any disciplinary action: oral warning, written warning and then dismissal. And it specificies possible reasons for summary dismissal: theft, drunkenness, illegal drug-taking and child abuse.

The contract requires the employer to specify the number of free days a week being offered, and the amount of paid holiday each year. The model contract also states that the employee will be be free on all Bank Holidays or will receive a day off in lieu. The employer undertakes to provide a pay slip on the day of payment, detailing gross payment, deductions and net payment.

The model contract for overseas nanny posts also includes a clause stating the employer's responsibility to pay the nanny's fares to and from the country. The employer is asked, among other points, to give details of the ages and gender of children, information on any other domestic staff, accommodation, any medical insurance offered and the location of the nearest British Consulate.

**Pay :**
Living-in Nanny – £120-£200 a week net.
Maternity Nurse living in – £250-£300 a week net.
Daily nanny/maternity nurse – £40 a day
Nanny working overseas – £150-£250 a week net

**Holidays:** 3-4 weeks

# 13 JOURNALISM AND PUBLIC RELATIONS

If you like variety, enjoy research and feel able to communicate with a large range of people you will find journalism very satisfying. You need to be able to cope with hassles and cut through bureaucracy, work under time pressures, and be able summarise complex issues in a readable way. The job also requires stamina and flexibility and you should be prepared to travel, sometimes at short notice. But it is rarely dull, and offers considerable scope for initiative. Journalists moan a lot but most would never seriously consider doing anything else. It is a wonderful career for the curious person, with a sense of humour, who hates hierarchies and routine.

You can apply direct to newspapers and magazines or go through a training scheme. About a dozen colleges offer one year pre-entry courses. Details from the National Council for the Training of Journalists (NCTJ). Courses for graduates are available at the City University, London, and the University of Wales, Cardiff. These courses include law, public affairs and shorthand.

The London College of Printing runs courses for people hoping to go into magazine journalism, covering reporting, interviewing, researching, sub-editing and word processing.

Many of these courses have well established links with employers and include a period of work experience on a newspaper or magazine. About 90 per cent of participants find jobs at the end, according to the NCTJ.

It is worth writing to publications you would like to work for, outlining your background and experience and asking if you could come in for a talk, even if no job is available at the moment. The editor may say no but keep your letter on file, or suggest some other publication which may be looking for staff. Much of journalism works through contacts and persistence pays off.

As a nurse you have a particular advantage in the specialist nursing and medical press. Both *Nursing Standard* and *Nursing Times* employ substantial numbers of nurses, and titles aimed at GPs, such as *Doctor, General Practitioner, Medical Monitor, Mims Magazine Weekly* and *Pulse* also look for people with a scientific background and understanding of the health service.

Several companies are now developing sponsored publications, paid for by pharmaceutical companies, and these also need journalists, sometimes on a freelance basis. Do not wait until a job is advertised before writing in. But always check and use the name of the editor.

## Freelance journalism

The Medical Journalists' Association includes more than 100 freelances, many of whom have moved on from full-time jobs in magazines and newspapers. Most undertake a variety of work including feature writing and conference reporting. Some contribute regular columns to women's magazines and newspapers, or produce newsletters for charities and drug companies. Many magazines employ freelances on a shift basis to cover sickness, holidays, maternity leave and sabbaticals. The successful freelance has a range of contacts, built up over several years, and a reputation for reliability.

But there is nothing to stop someone still in nursing from doing some freelance work, either as an adjunct to their full-time job or as a stepping stone to a job in journalism. Do not send articles in "on spec" but write first to the features editor, outlining your idea and asking if they are interested. The magazine may have carried something like

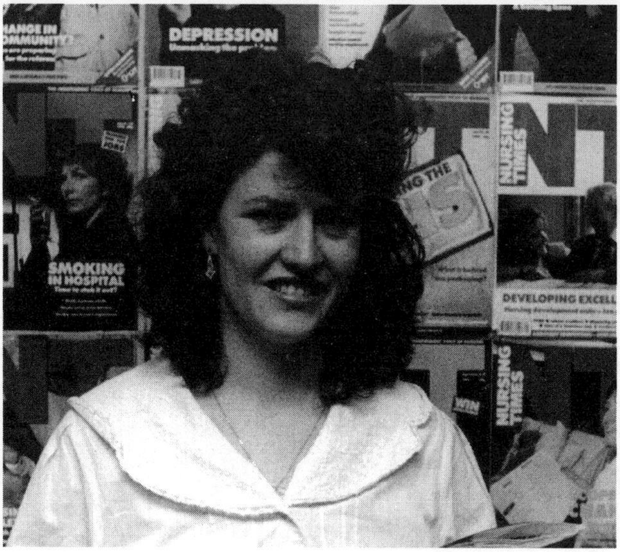


***Amanda Tattam**, aged 29, trained in Melbourne, and then went travelling working as a nanny, and then as a volunteer for CND. She joined Nursing Standard when it was launched in 1987 and now works as a reporter for Nursing Times.*

**“ My experience of journalism so far has been very good. I like the subject matter and enjoy digging out information and building up a story. I feel strongly that people must be made accountable.**

**I was a good nurse but I couldn’t stand the system and lack of support from seniors. It was not what I expected.**

**Journalism encourages you to question and you have to be able to ask total strangers extremely personal questions. It is more confrontational than nursing and there is less reverence for authority. As a journalist I am not afraid to talk to anybody. It is a very different culture but some of the skills needed – listening, empathy and good rapport with people – are the same as in nursing. And it is different every day. ”**

*After general and midwifery training in Wales and Sheffield,* ***June Thompson****, who is 48, spent 17 months in Lesotho, South Africa running a child health clinic at a Catholic mission hospital. She then trained as a health visitor and worked in Bangladesh and Papua New Guinea before returning to London, working as a health visitor and becoming editor of The Health Visitor magazine,a post she held for ten years. She is now a freelance journalist, contributing to women's magazines including Best, Prima and Everywoman, and the nursing press. She also writes reports for the Department of Health and books on child health.*

**" Journalism, and editing, are not as easy as I first thought. But the work is very enjoyable if you are curious and enjoy contact with people. I enjoy going to conferences and finding out what is going on.**

**And the empathy you develop as a nurse can be very helpful when doing interviews on distressing subjects. When a young mother with breast cancer broke down I think being a health visitor helped.**

**Now I like the freedom and variety of being freelance and I've never had to look for work. Going freelance after being in a job means you have to build up your reputation again. And it's very important to be reliable. But I wouldn't go back to a staff job. I work longer hours as a journalist than as a health visitor but it's less worrying. "**

it very recently, or have something in the pipeline.

Study the publication carefully, keep to whatever length is specified, and be prepared to rewrite your piece if requested. And don't expect overnight success. *Nursing Times* receives 40 features a week, of which 90 per cent are rejected.

Interest in health has increased enormously in the last

decade and the majority of the national newspapers now have a regular health page. Most rely heavily on pieces contributed by freelances. The editors of these pages are always on the look-out for ideas, particularly topical ones, and your nursing background can be an advantage.

When euthanasia is in the news, for example, an article on the ethical dilemmas for nurses could well be of interest. "First person" accounts, drawing on personal experience, have a perennial appeal. But find out the name of the person who edits the page, and ring or write before sending in your article.

**Pay:**
**Magazines**
Reporter specialist health magazine – £17,000- £18,000
Features editor, news editor, deputy editor – £23,000-£25,000
Editor – £35,000 plus car
Daily shift rate – £75-£120
Features, per 1,000 words – £100-£150

**Provincial Newspapers**
Trainees – £7,500-£12,000
Reporters/sub-editors – £12,000-£18,000

**National Newspapers**
Reporter/sub-editors – £35,000 plus
Features per 1,000 words – £200+
Freelance daily rate for journalists
working for public relations companies – £200-£300

**Holidays:** 4-6 weeks

# Public relations

Public relations is concerned with building up and maintaining favourable relationships between organisations and the public, including journalists, MPs, and consumers. The aim is to get the organisation, or product, known and

*After a four-year nursing degree at Chelsea College, London University, and a short spell in hospital nursing,* **Pamela Holmes** *went into a video production company and then into journalism, working as an editorial assistant on a computer magazine, sub-editor on Parents magazine and then as features editor on Nursing Times. She has also worked as a reporter for a medical TV company. Now 37, she is Press Officer for the Royal Free NHS Trust, Hampstead.*

**“ I enjoyed my degree but found nursing was not what I expected; at that time it didn't seem to offer much scope for initiative. But nursing gave me confidence and the ability to relate to people under stress which has stood me in good stead. As a press officer you have to be able to react quickly and deal with a large variety of people. You need to be calm under pressure and able to be objective. If there's a crisis you may have to organise a press conference at very short notice.**

**You have to understand how the organisation wants to put itself across, and try to give journalists what they need without disrupting the running of the hospital. That's not always easy, particularly with television crews. I take press calls, write press releases and patient information leaflets, and feed stories to the local press. I also produce a newsletter about the hospital for 1,900 local GPs for which I had to learn desk top publishing. I like being back in the NHS and part of a team which I admire. I feel I am doing something worthwhile and I enjoy working with people who really care. ”**

understood. The job involves planning programmes to put the organisation's aims or product across, writing press releases, making contacts with journalists, organising news conferences and product launches, producing company videos and newsletters, attending exhibitions and organising visits, receptions and corporate hospitality.

Not everyone in PR is a wild extravert but you do need to be able to get on with people, be sociable and diplomatic. You will need tact to balance your client's often unrealistic expectations with what is possible in terms of publicity, and keep a cool, objective head in times of crisis. Writing skills are also a necessity.

Some large organisations, such as the British Medical Association, Royal College of Nursing, health authorities and trusts employ their own "in house" PR officers while others use the services of a PR agency. Many do both. Some PR agencies serve a wide variety of clients while others specialise in the health field.

**Training**

There is no minimum educational entry requirement for public relations, although many entrants are graduates. Some agencies run their own training schemes. Courses are also provided by the Institute of Public Relations and the Public Relations Consultants Association,

Someone with a nursing background, able to offer knowledge of pharmacology and physiology and an understanding of the setting in which health professionals work, is at an advantage in agencies which specialise in pharmaceutical and health care work. But applicants without PR experience should be willing to go in at a fairly low level initially, and work their way up.

**PR Agencies**

The Public Relations Year Book, published by the Public Relations Consultants Association which claims to represent 85 per cent of the industry, lists the major agencies, their directors and clients. It is available in public libraries. Before writing to an agency on spec try to find out the name of the director of the health division, if any, or the personnel director.

Think about your own background and skills in terms of

***Averill Gordon,*** *aged 34, completed general nursing training in her native New Zealand before doing midwifery in Australia where she also specialised in intensive care. She has taught in a college of nursing, worked in corporate video production and completed a degree in English and mass communications. She worked at Shire Hall, a specialist healthcare agency, for 18 months as an account manager and is now an account director in the healthcare division of Burson-Marsteller, a large international public relations agency. Her principal clients are international pharmaceutical companies.*

**“ In PR you must give clients a feeling of competence and confidence. You must be a good listener, able to think quickly, and sociable. Initiative and being creative are also important. A nursing background helps because you already have time management skills, scientific knowledge and familiarity with the hospital hierarchy Part of my work is establishing groups of specialists in specific disease areas, to advise clients.**

**You do need tact, to educate clients into what is realistic. I find PR more stimulating than nursing but there is also more pressure. You can be in the office until midnight before a pitch for new business and then you have to be bright the next day.**

**It is quite a change in culture. Most nurses have low self-esteem but there is no place for that in an agency. Sometimes you can find the pursuit of profit a bit tedious. But I enjoy being responsible for budgets and seeing an idea through to fruition, and the work develops your confidence. But there is also insecurity. In PR you are only as good as your last project. Lose a client and your job could be in jeopardy. And the hours are quite long: 11 hour days are not unusual.**

**There is a lot of travel but I would not call it glamorous; there's usually no time to explore. ”**

what might be most useful in public relations. Stress any management or teaching experience, as well as research or writing projects you have undertaken. Public relations is primarily about communication so it is important to give a concise, interesting account of your experience.

The work of an in-house public relations officer includes writing press releases, organising press conferences, editing staff magazines, commissioning and organising exhibitions, arranging visits and liaising with politicians and civil servants as well as journalists.

It can be very satisfying work, particularly if you work for an organisation which practises or champions issues you regard as important. First contact should be by letter to the Personnel Director (by name) of the organisation you are interested in, enclosing a precise and interesting CV.

**Pay:**

**NHS Press Officers/Public Relations Officers**

Public relations assistant – £15,000
Public Relations Officer – £18,000-£20,000
Chief Public Relations Officer – £35,000
Press Officer NHS Trust, working alone – £20,000-£25,000
Press Officer, Royal College of Nursing – £24,000

Holidays: 6 weeks

**Public Relations Agencies**

Account Executive – £14,000-£15,000
Account Manager – £20,000-£25,000
Account Director – £40,000-£60,000
Managing Director – £60,000 plus

Holidays: 4-5 weeks

# 14 CONSULTANCY WORK

Being a consultant involves selling your own knowledge, expertise and experience. It can be done on a full or part-time basis, working as a one-person operation, or as part of a large consultancy employing hundreds of people. You may start out being asked to do small projects by contacts you make through your full-time job, and then decide to become a full-time consultant.

Whatever route you take, the work requires professional credibility, an entrepreneurial bent, logical thought, common sense, tact and the ability to write and present yourself well. You must become adept at identifying the client's needs, which may not always be immediately clear, and then agree a way of tackling them.

You must like people, and challenges. Consultants are often called in at moments of crisis or great change by organisations and individuals who feel they cannot deal with the current situation from their own resources. The approach to you, or your organisation, may be accompanied by a certain feeling of inadequacy, if not desperation.

In management consultancy you may find yourself called in to organisations or departments which have stopped functioning, where feelings of dissatisfaction and apprehension are running high. Part of your role will be to provide reassurance and restore confidence. And in Britain, with its tradition of reserve, that means listening to what is not said, as well as to what is, as management guru and former ICI Chairman, Sir John Harvey-Jones, has pointed out. Consultants should have good antennae and be quick on the uptake.

***David Rye**, aged 54, set up his own consultancy in 1987, specialising in management and organisational development work. He qualified as a nurse in 1967 and spent 10 years in clinical practice before going into nurse education. His previous posts include Director of Nurse Education for North West Surrey Health Authority, Director of Professional Activities at the Royal College of Nursing and Fellow at the King's Fund College. He is consultant editor of Senior Nurse.*

**" Networking and professional credibility are the most important aspects of being a consultant. If you are any good you don't need to do much marketing. I have established a client base of about 15 regular clients and the work comes in by personal recommendation and former colleagues.**

**Most of my work consists of identifying and solving problems, and running workshops with key managers. I was surprised, at first, at the ease with which the work came in.**

**Good "people" skills are important, and the ability to work in confidence. You also need to keep on top of the political agenda and have good business sense. The ability to diversify, and price yourself right, are also important. I usually spend three days a week in the field, and two at home, in the office.**

**I love the freedom of being a consultant, and the feeling of being in control. You get a lot of feedback and it's very rewarding. I earn twice as much as I did in a job. I think health authorities are becoming more cautious about using consultants, but there is plenty of work around. "**

Ideally you should be able to take sticky situations, and disarray, in your stride. A stable, pleasant, personality is certainly an asset. Flexibility is also important. Part of your success will depend on your ability to adapt to different working situations.

Consultants stress the importance of "knowing your niche" and this requires careful reflection on your experience, background and knowledge and examination of potential markets for them. This is important preparation. It is not enough to look good on paper, and show an impressive succession of jobs, unless you can convince potential clients that your particular skills can be tailored to meet their needs. All consultancy work involves a degree of self-promotion.

A high professional profile is certainly an advantage and the better you are known the less you have to market yourself. Setting yourself up as a consultant is unlikely to be viable early on in your career unless you have some rare and sought-after expertise. And in that case the consultancy work will probably come looking for you.

Most successful consultants seem to be in their middle or later years and have considerable experience. Age, allied to a determination to keep abreast, is an asset in this field.

## How to find work

The NHS's use of outside consultancy services has increased significantly in recent years, although just lately authorities have become more cautious. However the introduction of the internal market into the health service, and greater financial and managerial autonomy for hospitals, have increased the need for business and managerial skills.

Those experienced in implementing new patterns of work and re-organisations are particularly in demand.

Some of the large management consultancies, such as Price Waterhouse, employ senior nurses on their full-time staff, and also employ some on a contract basis for individual projects.

In the main, management consultancies require several

***Anne Palmer**, aged 42, spent 22 years in the NHS including seven years as senior tutor at St Mary's School of Nursing, Paddington, before starting her own education consultancy in 1991. She designed the curriculum outline for Nursing Times' Open Learning Programme and was involved in the preparation of demonstration districts for Project 2000. She lectures and organises workshops and conferences for hospitals, health authorities and colleges of higher education.*

**“ Being a consultant requires belief in yourself and keeping abreast of what is going on. It also involves quite a lot of groundwork before you start. It is important to look at your strengths and experience, research the market, find out what people are charging and get your pricing right.**

**You have to know your niche. Let people know that you are available and what you can offer. Networking is also important. You have to go to conferences and make sure you have your business cards.**

**You need adequate resources behind you: good clothes, a reliable car, computer, fax and answering machine. Computer skills are very useful. It also helps to have some capital behind you as payments can take several months to come in.**

**You need to be self-reliant and versatile and know how to pace yourself. Decide how many days a week you want to work and how much you can take on. Try and keep to set hours.**

**I believe in keeping in contact with other consultants in your field. If you cannot do a particular piece of work you can pass it on and someone else will do the same for you another time.**

**I also try to balance the time I spend out at conferences and workshops with working at home on longer-term research projects. ”**

years of experience at a managerial level and a good understanding of the NHS, and the healthcare field as a whole.

Information technology and computer skills are also an advantage as these are relatively new areas for the NHS. If you can offer experience, and contacts, at national or international level, so much the better.

If you plan to set up on your own, previous employers are one obvious source of potential business. Write to them pointing out that you are available and the sort of services you plan to offer. Report writing, advice on training packages, conferences, seminars, lectures, workshops, management development projects, research or whatever. Ask your contact to bear you in mind and pass the word round that you are available.

**Broaden your net**

Personal contacts are invaluable in bringing in business because they already know you and your work. But it is important to broaden your net all the time. Sending some promotional material – leaflets summarising your experience and what you are offering – will make it easier to circulate your details within the organisation.

Do not be afraid to break new ground and develop fresh outlets. That is part of the satisfaction of working as a consultant. If you have years of experience in a particular clinical area, for example, find out which publishers are producing books for that field and suggest yourself as a consultant/referee. The firm may also be looking for specialist input for new projects you do not know about.

If you have experience of computerised information systems being introduced into hospitals, you could suggest yourself as a part-time consultant to the suppliers, introducing the system to other units. Being a nurse, with hands-on experience of the system, you can add credibility to the operation and help allay staff wariness.

If you have worked at a fairly senior level in a clinical directorate, where specialists have taken over responsibility for their budget, your experience could be valuable in other hospitals undergoing similar changes.

As well as building up your own market and outlets it is important to be aware of what other consultants are up to. Some, quite naturally, may be very protective of their hard-won patch, and reluctant to tell you exactly what they do and charge. But others believe very strongly in sharing information and "low down", so you should be able to build up a picture of what to charge, the sort of work available, where opportunities are opening up, the good clients and the slow payers.

You should aim to build up an extensive network of fellow consultants as well as clients, so that you can pass on any work you are unable to take on and vice-versa. And this may not take as long as you first expect. Consultancy is very much about contacts.

**Pay:**

Senior Executive, Management Consultants
– £40,000-£50,000
Individual Self-Employed Consultants
in healthcare – £300-£500 per day

# 15 PART-TIME WORK AND JOB SHARING

Most of the occupations outlined in this book can be carried out on a part-time basis, and mainstream nursing is not short of opportunities for part-time work. About a third of the 320,000 nurses in the NHS are part-timers, working an average of 20 hours a week.

In addition to bank or agency nursing, and part-time nursing posts, several of the charities running helplines are willing to employ nurses on a part-time basis, and sometimes it is possible to work from home.

Nursing and residential homes, health clubs, complementary medicine clinics, general practice, occupational health nursing, journalism, public relations, consultancy and secretarial work are other possibilities.

Before looking for work you should analyse how much time you have available, how much you need to earn, whether and how far you are able to travel, and whether you want a regular commitment or the opportunity to pick and choose. It also helps to analyse your main reason for working. Money? To increase your long term career prospects? Stimulus?

Evidence from the NHS suggests that those in part-time posts are slow to be promoted. But moves are under way to change this. The NHS Management Executive has stated that by 1994 health authorities and trusts should ensure that all women returning to nursing after a career break or maternity leave, including part-timers and job sharers, should be able to go back at a grade equivalent to their leaving grade, and to work of a similar status.

The NHSME has also stated that all jobs should be

***Lesley Woodward, aged 36,*** *works as a breast care sister at Hull Royal Infirmary (HRI), working 18¾ hours a week as part of a job share. She is paid on G grade and has five weeks holiday a year. She trained at the HRI and worked for ten years, including five as part of a job share, as a district nursing sister, attached to a GP practice. She has two children. Her current job involves sitting in with the consultant when the diagnosis of breast cancer is given, following women up through their treatment and surgery, home visits, and introducing them to the cancer support group based at the hospital.*

**“ I wanted a job-share arrangement following the birth of my daughter five years ago and knew another district nursing sister who wanted to share. The health authority was reluctant initially because they thought it would threaten continuity of care. But we had a very supportive nursing officer and that helped. She drew up a rota with us and we had a three month trial. My current post was advertised as a job share.**

**I feel I have the best of both worlds – time for the children and an interesting job. I also have a leased car through the job which is a real perk. I couldn’t afford to run one if I didn’t work. My parents live nearby and my husband works from home so we have no childcare costs and my salary really makes a difference.**

**On the job front I find two heads are better than one and I get a lot of stimulus from the person I share with.**

**We are careful not to tread on each other’s space and try to keep our own caseloads. We work alternate days and some evenings and there is a good deal of flexibility. The person I work with has a grown up family and knows the pressures of juggling everything, and that is very helpful.**

**Good communication is essential if you are**

**considering a job share. In some ways I think you do a job twice as well when you are sharing because there is an added impetus to keep up the standard. I don't plan to go back to full-time work for some time and this arrangement gives me time to study as well.**

**I would advise anyone who wants to job share to find a potential partner and present yourselves to the health authority as a package. And offer to work on a trial basis for a time, if need be.** ”

offered on a job-share basis unless it can be shown that this is impossible. As part of the same drive the NHSME aims to increase the number of women in NHS general management posts from 18 per cent (1991) to 30 per cent by 1994.

## Part-time work

Part-time work offers a chance to get the feel of an organisation and may well lead to something permanent. You have a foot in the door and are in a good position to learn of any opportunities coming up.

When you have established the sort of hours you have available and the employment area you want to work in, study the relevant professional journals, national and local papers and contact local agencies. But do not leave it at that. Make as many contacts as possible and take the initiative.

Think of the exercise as promoting a valuable commodity – yourself – rather than scrambling for limited openings. If you would like to work for a particular organisation send your CV to the personnel director with a brief covering letter, outlining your skills and professional experience and saying you would be interested in working for them.

Employers are impressed by people who take the

initiative and you are likely to be borne in mind when something does come up. If you see a job you would like advertised, but cannot do it full time, apply anyway and ask if there is a possibility of doing it on a part-time or job-share basis. The employer may be willing to consider this, and you may be in a position to work more hours later on. At the very least you have made known your existence and availability.

## Job sharing

Research by the Institute of Manpower Studies at Sussex University and the Royal College of Nursing has shown that only about 200 nurses and midwives are working in job share arrangements in the NHS at the moment.

But there is nothing to stop you putting a job share proposition to a health authority or other employer. You probably stand the best chance if you can find a prospective sharer whose skills and availability complement your own . Then you can offer yourselves to an employer as a package And the organisation may well benefit from a broader range of experience and skill than one employee could be expected to offer.

**Points to consider**

- Each sharer should have their own written contract and job description
- Job sharers should work at least 16 hours a week to safeguard their entitlements to redundancy pay, maternity pay and maternity leave.
- Benefits should be spelt out at the outset. One office car, two or none?
- What happens if one sharer leaves? Will the employer advertise for a new "half" or will the remaining individual be redeployed or offered the post on a full-time basis?
- How will promotion work?

• Will your working week include any overlap period when you are both in the office or hospital together? Or will all communication between you be by telephone and notes?

Job sharing requires flexibility, compatibility, good communication and the ability to compromise, plus a willingness to share criticism as well as praise. The success of the arrangement will depend to a large extent on your rapport with the person you are sharing with. You must respect and trust each other even if your working methods do not coincide exactly.

You must be accountable to each other and make sure you always know what your other half has done. It is not for mavericks or loners or those with an overriding concern for personal advancement. The advantages are a regular pattern of work which allows for some flexibility, the benefits of being "on the staff' as well as having part of the week off, and the stimulus of having two minds on the job.

Guidance on job sharing is available from the Equal Opportunities Commission.

• **New Ways to Work**, a small London-based charity, provides information on flexible working hours, part-time work, career break schemes, job sharing and working from home. It also has a nursing job share contact list. The charity organises training and publishes a quarterly newsletter. Regional offices of the RCN also offer advice on job sharing and flexible working arrangements.

# 16 STARTING YOUR OWN BUSINESS / WORKING FROM HOME

Starting your own business can be all absorbing and very fulfilling. It will undoubtedly teach you a great deal, including enormous self-reliance, perseverance and resilience. But it is not for the faint-hearted or those who are reluctant to take responsibility. Almost all enterprises take more of your time, money and commitment than first envisaged.

You must be prepared for setbacks and ready to deal with the unexpected from the outset. You must also accept that there will be bad days. And very bad days. Getting out is not usually an option as your self-respect as well as your livelihood depend on success.

All self-employed people invest a great deal of themselves in their ventures, to a degree which is often hard to understand from the vantage point of a secure job. Working for yourself really is a different world and you should not take the plunge without research and reflection.

## Starting a business

Businesses are about buying and selling. To be successful you must find customers for your product or service who are prepared to a pay a price which makes it worth your while, not just today and tomorrow but in months and years to come. Obviously, demands, tastes and economic climates change, but you must research your potential market as well as possible, and preferably find some gap which you can fill. This may take the form of a new product, such as a newsletter for a group which has not previously had one, or a new/cheaper version of an established product or service.

### A business plan

It is important to prepare a business plan, particularly if you are hoping to borrow money. The plan should state what you intend to do and what resources are needed. It should describe your product or service and the potential markets for this, your competitors and your advantage over them. You should specify your needs in terms of equipment, staff and premises.

Most of the High Street banks provide advice packs on setting up in business, and the Federation of Small Businesses offers a free pack, *Be Your Own Boss.*

Advice is also available from local Training and Enterprise Councils (TECs – details from Job Centres and local telephone directories) which provide free help in preparing business plans, and also run courses and seminars.

TECs also provide financial help for new businesses. Conditions vary from area to area but allowances of £40-£60 a week are available for periods of 26 to 52 weeks during the first year of a new business. Some, but not all, schemes require you to have been unemployed for six weeks before applying and some require you to raise £1,000 of your own (or an overdraft facility) to put into the business.

### Value Added Tax

If your turnover comes to £37,600 or more in one year (1993-4 figures), you must register for Value Added Tax and charge VAT on all the goods and services you provide. Nursing and medical services are not generally subject to VAT. However, a nurse working as an osteopath, herbalist, chiropractor or acupuncturist, with a turnover of £37,600 or more, must charge VAT.

When invoicing you must add the current VAT rate to the bill for what you are supplying and fill in quarterly returns for the Customs and Excise Office. The procedure is time

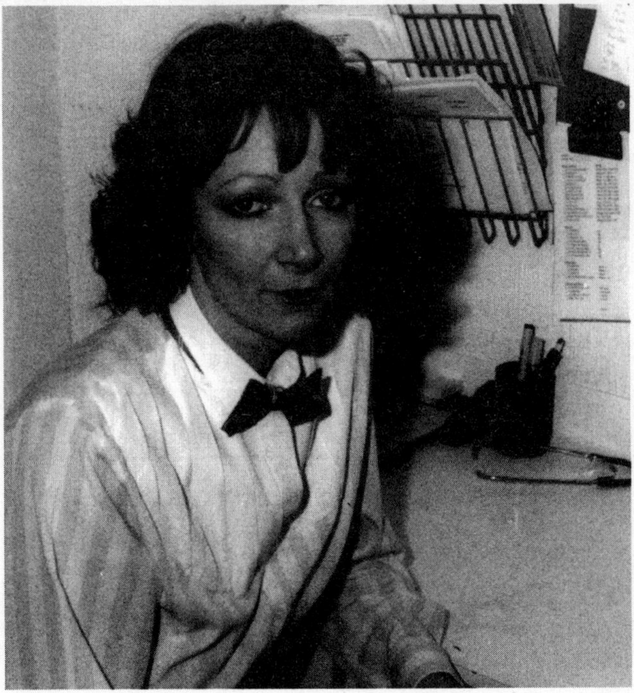

***Barbara Davies,** aged 38, trained at the Hammersmith hospital, London, worked in intensive care and cardiothoracic nursing and held a series of posts in private hospitals before setting up a nursing home for the Marie Stopes Clinic.*

*She started her own business in 1985, establishing the private Regents Park Clinic for sexually transmitted diseases, with a £15,000 bank loan and £5,000 of her own money. The clinic now employs a microbiologist, nurse/receptionist, eight doctors working on a sessional basis, and a part time book-keeper. It is open seven days a week and offers counselling and testing for all sexually transmitted diseases, including HIV, with results available on the same day, contraceptive services, pregnancy testing and abortion referral. Before opening the clinic Barbara spent a year in correspondence with the Department of Health to win a dispensation from the 1917 Venereal Disease Act which forbade advertising of a special clinic. She was gazumped four times when looking for premises and found landlords were reluctant to let to a new business.*

**" You never get bored running your own business and have a sense of achievement, and controlling your own destiny. You are always learning – marketing, advertising, personnel, administration and management.**

**But it can be very stressful. The first year I regretted ever having started. I was moonlighting six nights a week looking after an old lady in Belgravia because I needed the money, and working here during the day. My social life disappeared completely.**

**The rent was £10,000 a year and at one point I owed £30,000. I had a very helpful bank manager, and a consultation with a chartered accountant before I started who helped me draw up a business plan. But I did not appreciate how money just disappears like water into sand, however careful you are. Sometimes I had to pay the medical staff on Barclaycard.**

**Nursing training helps when running a business because you are taught to cope in a crisis and to organise your work and the people around you. It teaches you the importance of discipline and routine.**

**But it is very important to look after your health when you are working for yourself because you have forfeited the right to quit and can never go off sick. Now I make a reasonable living and get satisfaction from providing a good service.**

**The contact with patients is rewarding and I have learned an enormous amount about staff management. But you need to think carefully before starting up a business. You are manacled to it and that can induce claustrophobia. It's a love/hate relationship. "**

consuming, but not particularly difficult once you have the hang of it. Once registered you can reclaim the VAT you are charged on business expenses such as stationery, telephone bills, laywers' and accountants' fees. Local VAT offices are listed under Customs and Excise in telephone directories.

Once self-employed you will be responsible for your own national insurance contributions and tax. And you should think about paying into a pension scheme.

## Working from home

Freedom from commuting is not the only advantage of working at home. It is often possible to get more done without the distractions of colleagues and departmental upheavals. But you need to be self-disciplined, self-motivated and able to take a certain amount of isolation.

The flexibility and freedom which allow time to pick up children from school, and take some time off during the week when you have worked at the weekend, can all too easily eat into your working time so that you find you are not getting enough done. It is advisable to have some routine.

Factors to consider include:

- Space available. Do you have storage space as well as a quiet area where you can work?

- If customers/clients are coming to your house, can they be seen without going through your family rooms. If not, is this acceptable?

- Washing facilities: Can your washing machine cope with the extra towels from your treatment room. Or should you consider sending them to the laundry?

- Will you need extra insurance? Household insurance

policies do not always cover faxes and word processors.

• You will almost certainly need an answering machine. But how about an extra telephone line so business calls do not interrupt when you are "off duty"?.

On a more personal level, you need to consider the effect working at home will have on your social and family life. It can be difficult to shut the door at a certain hour and put it all behind you.

Those who work at home are considered to be both infinitely interruptible if there is a family crisis, and always available by customers and clients who do not have qualms about ringing up at odd hours. If you have only one phone line you may well get patients ringing up to discuss their symptoms while you are preparing Sunday lunch.

**Advice network**

If you are keen to make contact with others working at home you might consider joining Ownbase, whose network of some 400 members includes therapists, designers, translators, carers, financial advisers, photographers, consultants and people offering secretarial services. The association produces a newsletter and trading directory and offers a skills exchange, offering advice on topics such as printing and publicity. It also organises local meetings. Membership costs £17.50 a year.

# 17 DIRECTORY OF USEFUL CONTACTS AND ADDRESSES

## GENERAL PRACTICE

**Association of Medical Secretaries, Practice Administrators and Receptionists (AMSPAR)**
Tavistock House North
Tavistock Square
London WC1H 9LN
Tel: 071 387 6005
Fax: 071 388 2648

**Association of Health Centre and Practice Administrators**
Education Section
Berwyn
1 Oakmount Avenue
Chandlers Ford
Hampshire SO5 3AB
Tel: 0703 269372
Fax: 0703 269372

**English National Board for Nursing Midwifery and Health Visiting**
Resources and Careers Services
Woodseats House
764a Chesterfield Road
Sheffield S8 0SE
Tel: 0742 551064
Fax: 0742 555201

## OCCUPATIONAL HEALTH

**RCN Society of Occupational Health**
Royal College of Nursing
20 Cavendish Square
London W1M 0AB
Tel: 071 409 3333
Fax: 071 355 1379

**English National Board (Careers)**
PO Box 356
Sheffield S8 OSJ
Tel: 0742 555012
Fax: 0742 555201

## SCHOOL NURSING

**English National Board (Careers)**
PO Box 356
Sheffield S8 0SJ
Tel: 0742 555012
Fax: 0742 555201

**School Nurses Forum**
Royal College of Nursing
20 Cavendish Square
London W1M 0AB
Tel: 071 409 3333
Fax: 071 355 1379

## AGENCY WORK

**RCN Nursing Agencies Administrators Forum**
Royal College of Nursing
20 Cavendish Square
London W1M 0AB
Tel: 071 409 3333
Fax: 071 355 1379

**Allied Medicare Nursing Services**
Medicare House
Stone Business Park
Brooms Road
Stone
Staffordshire ST15 0TL
Tel: 0785 818914
Fax: 0785 818200

**British Nursing Association**
North Place
82 Great North Road
Hatfield
Hertfordshire AL9 5BL
Tel: 0707 263544
Fax: 0707 272250

**BUPA Nursing**
Fountain House
83 Fountain Street
Manchester M2 2BU
Tel: 061 228 7274
Fax: 061 236 5964

**London and Provincial Nursing Services**
76 Borough High Street
London SE1 1LL
Tel: 071 403 4693
Fax: 071 403 4320

**Reed Nurse**
193 Victoria Street
London SW1E 5NE
Tel: 071 828 8625
Fax: 071 630 5030

## PHARMACEUTICAL INDUSTRY

**Association of Clinical Pharmacology Nurses**
Chair/secretary:
Penny Thorne
Clinical Unit Manager
Smith Kline & Beecham
Coldharbour Road
The Pinnacles
Harlow
Essex CM19 5AD
Tel: 0279 622000
Fax: 0279 622100

**Innovex Ltd.**
309 Reading Road
Henley-on-Thames
Oxfordshire RG9 1EL
Tel: 0491 578171

Fax: 0491 575057
(Recruitment agency which also does contract work for pharmaceutical industry)

**Association of British Pharmaceutical Industry**
12 Whitehall
London SW1A 2DY
Tel: 071 930 3477
Fax: 071 930 3290

**MIMS (Monthly Index of Medical Specialties)**
30 Lancaster Gate
London W2 3LP
Tel: 081 943 5000
Fax: 071 413 4066
Includes list of drug companies

## COUNSELLING, CHIROPODY, PHYSIOTHERAPY, SOCIAL WORK

**British Association for Counselling**
1 Regent Place
Rugby CV21 2PJ
Tel: 0788 550899
Information: 0788 578328
Fax: 0788 562189

**National Association for Staff Support**
9 Caradon Close
Woking
Surrey GU21 3DU
Tel: 0483 771599

**The Society of Chiropodists**
53 Welbeck Street
London W1M 7HE
Tel: 071 486 3381
Fax: 071 935 6359

**Council for Professions Supplementary to Medicine**
Park House
184 Kennington Park Road
London SE11 4BU
Tel: 071 582 0866
Fax: 071 820 9684

**The Chartered Society of Physiotherapy**
14 Bedford Row
London WC1R 4ED
Tel: 071 242 1941
Fax: 071 831 4509

**Therapy Weekly**
4 Little Essex Street
London WC2R 3LF
Tel: 071 836 6633
Fax: 071 836 0798

**Central Council for Education and Training in Social Work**
Derbyshire House
St Chad's Street
London WC1H 8AD
Tel: 071 278 2455
Fax: 071 278 2934

**Community Care**
14th Floor, Quadrant
House, Sutton
Surrey SM2 5AS
Tel: 081 652 4861
Fax: 081 652 4739

**COMPLEMENTARY THERAPIES**

**Complementary Therapies in Nursing Special Interest Group**
Royal College of Nursing
20 Cavendish Square
London W1M OAB
Tel: 071 409 3333
Fax: 071 355 1379

**Council for Acupuncture**
179 Gloucester Place
London NW1 6DX
Tel: 071 724 5756

**British Acupuncture Association**
8 Hunter Street
London WC1N 1BN
Tel: 071 833 8164

**Aromatherapy Organisations Council**
3 Latymer Close
Braybrooke
Market Harborough
Leicestershire LE16 8LN
Tel: 0455 615466
Fax: 0455 615054

**International Federation of Aromatherapists**
Department of Continuing Education
The Royal Masonic Hospital
Ravenscourt Park
London W6 0TN
Tel: 081 846 8066

**British Chiropractic Association**
29 Whitley Street
Reading
Berkshire RG2 0EG
Tel: 0734 757557
Fax: 0734 757257

**Anglo-European College of Chiropractic**
Parkwood Road
Bournemouth BH5 2DF
Tel: 0202 431021
Fax: 0202 417352

**National Institute of Medical Herbalists**
9 Palace Gate
Exeter
Devon EX1 1JA
Tel: 0392 426022

**The School of Phytotherapy (Herbal Medicine)**
Bucksteep Manor
Bodle Street Green
Hailsham
East Sussex BN27 4RJ
Tel: 0323 833812

**The Society of Homeopaths**
2 Artizan Road
Northampton NN1 4HU
Tel: 0604 21400

**London College of Massage**
5-6 Newman Passage
London W1P 3PF
Tel: 071 323 3574
Fax: 071 436 9618

**Northern Institute of Massage**
100 Waterloo Road
Blackpool FY4 1AW
Tel: 0253 403548

**General Council and Register of Osteopaths**
56 London Street
Reading
Berkshire RG1 4SQ
Tel: 0734 576585
Fax: 0734 566246

**Osteopathic Information Service**
Munro and Forster PR
37 Soho Square
London W1V 5DG
Tel: 071 439 7177
Fax: 071 437 0553

**British School of Naturopathy and Osteopathy**
6 Netherhall Gardens
London NW3 5RR
Tel: 071 435 6464
Fax: 071 431 3630

**British School of Osteopathy**
1-4 Suffolk Street
London SW1Y 4HG
Tel: 071 930 9254
Fax: 071 839 1098

**European School of Osteopathy**
104 Tonbridge Road
Maidstone
Kent ME16 8SL
Tel: 0622 671558
Fax: 0622 662165

**British Reflexology Association**
Monks Orchard
Whitbourne
Worcester WR6 5RB
Tel/Fax: 0886 21207

**British Complementary Medicine Association**
Exmoor Street
London W10 6DZ
Tel: 081 964 1205
Fax: 081 964 1207

**Institute for Complementary Medicine**
PO Box 194
London SE16 1QZ
Tel: 071 237 5165
Fax: 071 237 5175

**International Therapy Examination Council**
James House
Oaklebrook Mill
Newent
Gloucestershire GL18 1HD
Tel: 0531 821875
Fax: 0531 822425

## WORKING IN TRAVEL & NURSING ABROAD

**Thomson Tour Operations**
Overseas Personnel Department
Greater London House
Hampstead Road
London NW1 7SD
Tel: 071 387 9321
Fax: 071 387 8451

**Alternative Travel Group**
69-71 Banbury Road
Oxford OX2 6PE
Tel: 0865 310399
Fax: 0865 310299

**The Independent Guide to Real Holidays Abroad**
The Independent
40 City Road
London EC1Y 2DB
Tel: 071 253 1222
Fax: 071 956 1453

**Inflight Nurses Association**
Royal College of Nursing
20 Cavendish Square
London W1M 0AB
Tel: 071 409 3333
Fax: 071 355 1379

**Europ Assistance**
252 High Street
Croydon
Surrey CRO 1NF
Tel: 081 680 1234
Fax: 081 680 8992

**Travellers' Medical Services**
Golden Square
Petworth
West Sussex GU28 0AP
Tel: 0798 44042
Fax: 0798 42164

**Trans-Care International**
193 High Street
Acton
London W3 9DD
Tel: 081 993 6151
Fax: 081 993 8334

**International Assistance Services**
32 High Street
Purley
Surrey CR8 2PP
Tel: 081 763 1550
Fax: 081 643 7735

**Institute of Advanced Nursing Education**
Royal College of Nursing
20 Cavendish Square
London W1M 0AB

Tel: 071 872 0840
Fax: 071 355 1379

**British Airways Medical Services for Travellers Abroad (BAMSTA)**
7 Bury Place
London WC1A 2LA
Tel: 071 831 3266
Fax: 071 430 1637

**Cunard Line**
South Western House
Canute Road
Southampton SO9 1ZA
Tel: 0703 229933
Fax: 0703 225843

**P & O Cruises**
Dukes Keep
Marsh Lane
Southampton SO9 4GU
Tel: 0703 336262
Fax: 0703 227920

**AMI Middle East Services**
7/9 St James's Street
London SW1A 1EE
Tel: 071 839 3812
Fax: 071 973 0278

**Arabian Careers Ltd.**
115 Shaftesbury Avenue
London WC2H 8AD
Tel: 071 379 7877
Fax: 071 379 0885

**International Hospitals Group**
Stoke Park
Stoke Poges
Slough SL2 4NS
Tel: 0753 573222
Fax: 0753 535855

**GAMA International**
2nd Floor
Moreau House
116 Brompton Road
London SW3 1JJ
Tel: 071 581 5544
Fax: 071 581 8544

**United Medical Enterprises**
21 Manchester Square
London W1M 5AD
Tel: 071 224 2900
Fax: 071 935 4377

**International Health Exchange**
Africa Centre
38 King Street
London WC2E 8JT
Tel: 071 836 5833
Fax: 071 379 1239

**Voluntary Sevices Overseas**
317 Putney Bridge Road
London SW15 2PN
Tel: 081 780 2266
Fax: 081 780 1326

**CIIR - Catholic Institute for International Relations**
Unit 3
Canonbury Yard
190A New North Road

London N1 7BJ
Tel: 071 354 0883
Fax: 071 359 0017

**Save the Children Fund**
17 Grove Lane
London SE5 8RD
Tel: 071 703 5400
Fax: 071 703 2278

**NHS Overseas Enterprises**
3 Craven Hill
London W2 3EN
Tel: 071 224 9091
Fax: 071 224 9044

**Raleigh International**
Alpha Place
Flood Street
London SW3 5SZ
Tel: 071 351 7541
Fax: 071 351 9372

**BUNACAMP**
**BUNAC**
16 Bowling Green Lane
London EC1R OBD
Tel: 071 251 3472
Fax: 071 251 0215

**Royal College of Nursing International Office**
RCN
20 Cavendish Square
London W1M OAB
Tel: 071 409 3333
Fax: 071 355 1379

**WORKING FOR A CHARITY**

**BACUP – British Association of Cancer United Patients**
3 Bath Place
Rivington Street
London EC2A 3JR
Tel: 071 696 9003
Fax: 071 696 9002

**CancerLink**
17 Britannia Street
London WC1X 9JN
Tel: 071 833 2451
Fax: 071 833 4963

**CancerLink Scotland**
9 Castle Terrace
Edinburgh EH1 2DP
Tel: 031 228 5557
Fax: 031 228 6710

**Medical Advisory Service**
10 Barley Mow Passage
London W4 4PH
Tel: 081 994 9874
Fax: 081 995 0113

**British Diabetic Association**
10 Queen Anne Street
London W1M 0BD
Tel: 071 323 1531
Fax: 071 637 3644

**British Heart Foundation**
14 Fitzhardinge Street

London W1H 4DH
Tel: 071 935 0185
Fax: 071 486 5820

**Multiple Sclerosis Society**
25 Effie Road
London SW6 1EE
Tel: 071 736 6267
Fax: 071 736 9861

**National Asthma Campaign**
Providence House
Providence Place
London N1 ONT
Tel: 071 226 2260
Fax: 071 704 0740

**National Osteoporosis Society**
PO Box 10
Radstock
Bath BA3 3YB
Tel: 0761 432472
Fax: 0761 437903

## NURSING HOMES AND RESIDENTIAL CARE HOMES

**RCN Association for Care of the Elderly (ACE), and**

**RCN Residential Care Managers Special Interest Group**
Royal College of Nursing
20 Cavendish Square
London W1M 0AB
Tel: 071 409 3333
Fax: 071 355 1379

**Registered Nursing Homes Association**
Calthorpe House
Hagley Road
Edgbaston
Birmingham B16 8QY
Tel: 021 454 2511
Fax: 021 454 0932

**British Federation of Care Home Proprietors**
852 Melton Road
Thurmaston
Leicester LE4 8BN
Tel: 0533 640095
Fax: 0533 640141

**National Care Home Association**
5 Bloomsbury Place
London WC1A 2QA
Tel: 071 436 1871
Fax: 071 436 1193

**Independent Healthcare Association**
22 Little Russell Street
London WC1A 2HT
Tel: 071 430 0537
Fax: 071 242 2681

**Care Concern** *(journal for nursing and residential home owners/managers)*
Hawker Publications Ltd

13 Park House
140 Battersea Park Road
London SW11 4NB
Tel: 071 720 2108
Fax:071 498 3023

**English National Board (Careers)**
Woodseats House
764A Chesterfield Road
Sheffield S8 OSE
Tel: 0742 551064
Fax: 0742 555201

## WORKING AS A NANNY

**Federation of Recruitment and Employment Services (FERES)**
36-38 Mortimer Street
London W1N 7RB
Tel: 071 323 4300
Fax: 071 255 2878

**Kensington Nannies**
49-53 Kensington High St
London W8 5ED
Tel: 071 937 2333
Fax: 071 937 1027

**Nannies Incorporated**
*(offices in Brussels and Paris)*
18B Princes Place
Holland Park
London W11 4QA
Tel: 071 229 1214
Fax: 071 229 6558

**Nannies International**
14-16 Hoghton Street
Southport PR9 OPA
Tel: 0704 546153
Fax: 0704 501092

**Occasional and Permanent Nannies**
2 Cromwell Place
London SW7 2JE
Tel: 071 225 1555
Fax: 071 589 4966

**Playtime**
90 Grandison Road
London SW121 6LN
Tel: 071 673 3433

**Tate International**
(specialises in Italy)
Southbank House
Black Prince Road
London SE1 9SJ
Tel: 071 793 0406
Fax: 071 587 0988

**Universal Aunts**
PO Box 304
London SW4 ONN
Tel: 071 738 8937
Fax: 071 622 1914

**The Lady**
40 Bedford Street
WC2E 9EN
Tel: 071 379 4717
Fax: 071 497 2137

**Nursery World**
51 Calthorpe Street
London WC1X OHH
Tel: 071 837 7224
Fax: 071 278 3896

**Nursing Times**
4 Little Essex Street
London WC2R 3LF
Tel: 071 379 0970
Fax: 071 497 266

**JOURNALISM AND PUBLIC RELATIONS WORK**

**National Council for the Training of Journalists**
Latton Bush Centre
Southern Way
Harlow
Essex CM18 7BL
Tel: 0279 430009
Fax: 0279 438008

**City University**
Northampton Square
London EC1V 0HB
Tel: 071 477 8000
Fax: 071 477 8560

**Centre for Journalism Studies**
University of Wales
69 Park Place
Cardiff CF1 3AS
Tel: 0222 874000
Fax: 0222 371921

**London College of Printing**
Elephant and Castle
London SE1 6SB
Tel: 071 735 8484
Fax: 071 587 5297

**Nursing Standard**
Viking House
17-19 Peterborough Road
Harrow
Middlesex HA1 2AX
Tel: 081 423 1066
Fax: 081 423 6570

**Nursing Standard** also publishes **Senior Nurse, Paediatric Nursing and Nursing the Elderly.**

**Nursing Times**
Macmillan Magazines
4 Little Essex Street
London WC2R 3LF
Tel: 071 379 0970
Fax: 071 497 2664

Macmillan also publishes **Community Outlook, The Health Service Journal** and **Therapy.**

**Doctor**
Reed Business Publishing
Quadrant House
The Quadrant
Sutton
Surrey SM2 5AS

Tel: 081 652 3500
Fax: 081 652 8701

Reed also publishes **Hospital Doctor and Practice Nurse**

**General Practitioner**
Haymarket Publishing
30 Lancaster Gate
London W2 3LP
Tel: 081 943 5000
Fax: 071 413 4513

Haymarket also publishes **MIMS, MIMS Magazine Weekly, Fundholding, Medeconomics** and **GP Nurse Today.**

**Medical Monitor**
Medicom
118 London Road
Kingston-upon-Thames
Surrey KT2 6QJ
Tel: 081 541 5666
Fax: 081 541 4746

Medicom also publishes **Horizons, Management in General Practice** and **Healthcare Management**

**Pulse**
Morgan-Grampian Publications
30 Calderwood Street
London SE18 6BQ
Tel: 081 855 7777
Fax: 081 855 2406

Morgan-Grampian also publishes **The Practitioner**

**Professional Nurse**
Brook House
2-16 Torrington Place
London WC1E 7LT
Tel: 071 636 4622
Fax: 071 637 3021

**British Journal of Nursing**
Mark Allen Publishing Ltd.
Croxted Mews
288 Croxted Road
London SE24 9BY
Tel: 081 671 7521
Fax: 081 671 7327

Mark Allen also publishes **Practice Nursing** and **British Journal of Hospital Medicine**

**The Medical Journalists Association**
Secretary - Mrs Gwen Yates
Old Barley Mow
185 High Street
Stony Stratford
Milton Keynes MK11 1AP
Tel: 0908 564623

**The Public Relations Consultants Association**
Willow House

Willow Place
London SW1P 1JH
Tel: 071 233 6026
Fax: 071 828 4797

**The Institute of Public Relations**
The Old Trading House
15 Northburgh Street
London EC1V 0PR
Tel: 071 253 5151
Fax: 071 490 0588

**National Association of Health Service Public Relations Officers (NAHSPRO)**
Chairman - Linda Rolf
Public Relations Manager
South West Thames
Regional Health Authority
40 Eastbourne Terrace
London W2 3QR
Tel: 071 725 2500
Fax: 071 258 3908

## SPECIALIST HEALTHCARE PR AGENCIES

**Brandon Harris & Company**
Suite 201a
Butlers Wharf
45 Curlew Street
London SE1 2ND
Tel: 071 407 6854
Fax: 071 407 7218

**Counsellor**
Brands House
Kingshill Road
Four Ashes
High Wycombe
Bucks HP13 5BB
Tel: 0494 711228
Fax: 0494 716626

**Fusion Communications**
227-229 Chiswick High Rd
London W4 2DW
Tel: 081 747 8797
Fax: 081 747 8977

**Henderson Group One**
1 Roberts Mews
Lowndes Place
London SW1X 8DA
Tel: 071 235 4086/7

**Ryde House**
Ripley
Surrey GU23 6AT
Tel: 0483 225398
Fax: 0483 211043

**Magellan Medical Communications**
40-42 Osnaburgh Street
London NW1 3ND
Tel: 071 465 8366
Fax: 071 465 8367

**Medical Action Communications**
Action International House
Crabtree Office Village

Eversley Way
Thorpe
Egham
Surrey TW20 8RY
Tel: 0784 434353
Fax: 0784 431323

**MC2: Medical & Media Communications**
Brigade House
8 Parsons Green
London SW6 4TN
Tel: 071 371 5044
Fax: 071 371 8432

**Medical Viewpoint**
The Old Ribbon Mill
Pitt Street
Macclesfield
Cheshire SK11 7PT
Tel: 0625 618507
Fax: 0625 610260

**Shire Hall**
3 Olaf Street
London W11 4BE
Tel: 071 229 9922
Fax: 071 229 2989

**Vox Prism**
Pinewood Studios
Iver Heath
Buckinghamshire SLO ONH
Tel: 0753 631033
Fax: 0753 630435

## AGENCIES WITH A HEALTHCARE DIVISION

**Burson-Marsteller**
24 Bloomsbury Way
London WC1A 2PX
Tel: 071 831 6262
Fax: 071 430 1033

**Edelman Public Relations**
Kingsgate House
536 Kings Road
London SW10 0TE
Tel: 071 835 1222
Fax: 071 351 7676

**Fleishman-Hillard**
25 Wellington Street
London WC2E 7DA
Tel: 071 306 9000
Fax: 071 497 0096

**Ketchum Public Relations**
5 Langley Street
WC2H 9JA
Tel: 071 379 3404
Fax: 071 240 8311

**Hill and Knowlton**
5-11 Theobalds Road
London WC1X 8SH
Tel: 071 413 3000
Fax: 071 413 3111

**Manning Selvage & Lee**
199 Knightsbridge
London SW7 1RP
Tel: 071 823 9666
Fax: 071 823 8089

**The Rowland Company**
67 Whitfield Street
London W1P 5RL
Tel: 071 436 4060
Fax: 071 255 2131

## CONSULTANCY WORK

**TENDA - The European Nursing Development Agency**
Tameside General Hospital
Fountain Street
Ashton-under-Lyne
Lancashire OL6 9RW
Tel: 061 339 5535
Fax: 061 339 5512

**Arthur Andersen**
1 Surrey Street
London WC2R 2PS
Tel: 071 438 3000
Fax: 071 831 1133

**Coopers & Lybrand**
Plumtree Court
London EC4A 4HT
Tel: 071 583 5000
Fax: 071 822 4652

**PA Consulting Group**
123 Buckingham Palace Road
London SW1W 9SR
Tel: 071 730 9000
Fax: 071 733 5040

**Price Waterhouse**
32 London Bridge Street
London SE1 9SY
Tel: 071 939 3000
Fax: 071 378 0647

**National Health Service Training Directorate**
St Bartholomew's Court
18 Christmas Street
Bristol BS1 5BT
Tel: 0272 291029
Fax: 0272 250574

## PART TIME WORK & JOB SHARING

**Equal Opportunities Commission**
Overseas House
Quay Street
Manchester M3 3HN
Tel: 061 833 9244
Fax: 061 835 1657

**New Ways to Work**
309 Upper Street
London N1 2TY
Tel: 071 226 4026

**NHS Women's Unit (part of the NHS Management Executive)**
Room 1002
Hannibal House
Elephant & Castle
London SE1 6TE
Tel: 071 972 2078
Fax: 071 972 1448

**Part Time Careers Ltd**
10 Golden Square
London W1R 3AF
Tel: 071 437 3103/734 0559
Fax: 071 494 1154

## STARTING YOUR OWN BUSINESS & WORKING FROM HOME

**Federation of Small Businesses**
140 Lower Marsh
Westminster Bridge
London SE1 7AE
Tel: 071 928 9272
Fax: 071 401 2544

**Ownbase**
68 First Avenue
Bush Hill Park
Enfield EN1 1BN
Tel/Fax: 081 363 0808

**Training and Enterprise Education Directive**
Moorfoot
Sheffield S1 4PQ
Tel: 0742 753275
Fax: 0742 758316

**VAT Central Unit**
Alexander House
21 Victoria Avenue
Southend on Sea SS99 1AA
Tel: 0702 348944
Fax: 0702 366085

# INDEX OF CAREERS